AF779943

Application of Cone Beam Computed Tomography for Maxillofacial Diseases

Application of Cone Beam Computed Tomography for Maxillofacial Diseases

Guest Editor

Yiu Yan Leung

MDPI

Basel • Beijing • Wuhan • Barcelona • Belgrade • Novi Sad • Cluj • Manchester

Guest Editor
Yiu Yan Leung
Faculty of Dentistry
The University of Hong Kong
Hong Kong
China

Editorial Office
MDPI AG
Grosspeteranlage 5
4052 Basel, Switzerland

This is a reprint of the Special Issue, published open access by the journal *Diagnostics* (ISSN 2075-4418), freely accessible at: https://www.mdpi.com/journal/diagnostics/special_issues/08P847QJXQ.

For citation purposes, cite each article independently as indicated on the article page online and as indicated below:

Lastname, A.A.; Lastname, B.B. Article Title. *Journal Name* **Year**, *Volume Number*, Page Range.

ISBN 978-3-7258-7502-3 (Hbk)
ISBN 978-3-7258-7503-0 (PDF)
https://doi.org/10.3390/books978-3-7258-7503-0

© 2026 by the authors. Articles in this reprint are Open Access and distributed under the Creative Commons Attribution (CC BY) license. The reprint as a whole is distributed by MDPI under the terms and conditions of the Creative Commons Attribution-NonCommercial-NoDerivs (CC BY-NC-ND) license (https://creativecommons.org/licenses/by-nc-nd/4.0/).

Contents

About the Editor

Yiu Yan Leung

Yiu Yan Leung serves as a Clinical Professor and Postgraduate Programme Director in Oral and Maxillofacial Surgery at the Faculty of Dentistry, University of Hong Kong. Additionally, he holds the position of Associate Dean (Global Engagement and Development) of the Faculty. Prof. Leung is also the President of the Hong Kong Association of Oral and Maxillofacial Surgeons (2022–2026) and the President of the Asian Association of Oral and Maxillofacial Surgeons (2024–2026).

After graduating with a BDS, MDS (OMFS), and PhD from the University of Hong Kong, Prof. Leung began his career in oral and maxillofacial surgery in Hong Kong. With over 150 publications in peer-reviewed international journals, he ranks among the Top 2% of the World's Most Cited Scientists by Stanford University for 2021–2024. Prof. Leung's clinical and research interests encompass orthognathic surgery, management of obstructive sleep apnea, temporomandibular disorder, trigeminal nerve repair, and management of complications after dentoalveolar surgery. As a renowned expert in his field, he frequently delivers lectures both regionally in the Asia Pacific and internationally.

diagnostics

MDPI

Article

Evaluation of Root Canal Configuration of Maxillary and Mandibular First Molar by CBCT: A Retrospective Cross-Sectional Study

Rakan Rafdan Alhujhuj, Rizwan Jouhar *, Muhammad Adeel Ahmed, Abdullatif Abdulrahman Almujhim, Mohammed Tariq Albutayh and Necdet Adanir

Department of Restorative Dental Sciences, College of Dentistry, King Faisal University, Al-Ahsa 31982, Saudi Arabia
* Correspondence: rjouhar@kfu.edu.sa; Tel.: +966-59-3114621

Abstract: Adequate knowledge of root canal morphology along with its probable variations is imperative to acquire successful endodontic treatment. This retrospective cross-sectional study aimed to investigate the root canal configuration of maxillary and mandibular first molar using Cone-Beam Computed Tomography (CBCT) among patients in Al-Ahsa region, Saudi Arabia. A total of 377 samples were included, out of which 123 CBCT (I-CAT Vision QTM) scans with intact all first permanent molars were selected in this study and scanned in sagittal, axial, and coronal views by using BlueSkyPlan software. The number of canals in each root and their configuration according to the Vertucci classification system was evaluated. Statistical analysis was analyzed using SPSS version 21 (IBM). Chi-square test was applied to evaluate the association of root canal morphology and mandibular and maxillary first molars with respect to gender. Out of 123 CBCT scans, 59 (48.0%) were males and 64 (52.0%) were females; the mean age was 26.95 ± 10.65 years. The mesiobuccal root of bilateral maxillary first molar had Type-I (87.0%) of Vertucci classification followed by Type-IV (9.8%). Additionally, all mesiobuccal roots (100%) of the left mandibular first molar had Type-I of Vertucci's classification. A significant association has been observed between gender and a number of canals in bilateral maxillary first molars. Females showed a significantly higher prevalence of three-root canal configuration in maxillary first molars of both sides compared four canals found most commonly in males ($p = 0.004$). This study concluded that the majority of maxillary and mandibular permanent first molars had three roots and three canals with Type-I Vertucci's classification in patients belonging to the Al-Ahsa region of the Saudi Arabia. It was also proved that gender is significantly associated with the number of canals in a bilateral maxillary molar.

Keywords: cone-beam computed tomography; endodontics; maxillary first molar; mandibular first molar; root canal configuration; Vertucci's classification

1. Introduction

Knowledge of root canal morphology is key to practicing successful endodontic treatment. The occurrence of anatomical variations in the root canal system has always been a leading endodontic challenge to dental practitioners [1].

Endodontic treatment includes cleaning and shaping of root canals, elimination of inflamed or necrotic pulp tissues and subsequently obturation of prepared canals [2]. Failure of endodontic treatment has various reasons, one of which is undetected or missed canals due to complex morphology [3]. Untreated root canals act as reservoirs for bacterial growth which eventually leads to treatment failure [4–6].

Vertucci [7] has categorized root canal anatomical patterns of permanent teeth into eight types. Hasan et al. [8] reported that unsuccessful endodontic treatment of maxillary teeth was associated with inappropriate detection and treatment of all canals, particularly the second mesiobuccal canal (MB2). Consequently, dental practitioners must be familiar with probable structural deviation. It has been predicted by some researchers who considered the morphology of maxillary first molar that most cases reported a higher frequency of a second mesiobuccal root (MBR) canal [9]. Similarly, Abd-Latib et al. [10] conducted a study in Malaysia, observing the high prevalence of MB2 canal in maxillary first molar specifically in males. Furthermore, another study reported the prevalence of MB2 canal in 55.8% cases of studied maxillary molars [11]. Likewise, AL-Alawi et al. reported a 4.9% occurrence of radix molars after extraction amongst Malaysians, however radix entomolaris (4.3%) was more prevalent as compared to radix paramolaris (0.3%) [12]. Many researchers have evaluated the morphology of mandibular first molars root canal with respect to the genders and race, where conventional two-dimensional (2D) periapical radiograph and demineralization-staining techniques were used [13,14].

Cone-beam computed tomography (CBCT) is used as a dental diagnostic tool [15,16]. It presents high-quality three-dimensional information and has been shown to be a better technique for pretreatment evaluation of root canal morphology [17]. CBCT is one of the advanced imaging modalities that is capable of overwhelming the superimposition of adjacent structures, and its three-dimensional property makes it superior to conventional periapical radiography [18]. This radiographic modality permits investigation to be done without devastation of tissues and allows normal functioning of natural teeth in the oral cavity.

Studies among the Saudi Arabian sub-population by Al-Fouzan et al. [19] and Alrahabi et al. [20] investigated the morphology of the permanent maxillary first molars by using CBCT (in vitro) and conventional radiographs (in vivo). They showed prevalence of two canals in the MBR estimated as 70.6% in vitro and ranging from 23.3% to 51.3% in vivo. Many researchers have established the superior effect of high-quality three-dimensional images by CBCT over conventional radiographic techniques, in order to study the morphology of root canal system [21–23]. CBCT is believed to be an effective adjunctive diagnostic tool that assists in dealing with management, diagnosis, and follow-up [24]. It reflects the accurate similar results that can be obtained by using modified staining techniques and tooth sectioning to identify the variation in root canal morphology [25,26].

Al-Ahsa is in the southeastern part of the Kingdom of Saudi Arabia, where it occupies the southern part of the Eastern Province. It covers a large area of about 530 thousand square kilometers, representing 68% of the Eastern Region and 24% of the Kingdom. The population of Al-Ahsa is over one million. Al-Ahsa is an agricultural oasis embodied by the nature of the place and the abundance of water. There are more than two million palm trees in Al-Ahsa; these trees produce the best types of dates in the world.

Comprehensive information of the most common root and root canal morphologies with their variations is imperative to support dental practitioners in identifying irregularities during root canal therapy to increase successful outcome. To the best of our knowledge, there is no study conducted to explore the root canal morphology of maxillary and mandibular first molars in the Al-Ahsa region of Saudi Arabia. The aim of the current study was to investigate the root canal configuration of maxillary and mandibular first molar using Cone-Beam Computed Tomography (CBCT) in patients belonging to the Al-Ahsa region of Saudi Arabia.

2. Materials and Methods

This retrospective cross-sectional study was conducted at Dental Complex of King Faisal University after obtaining ethical approval from the Research Ethics Committee of Deanship of Scientific Research at King Faisal University (KFU-REC/2020-10-21). Data were collected from digitized CBCT images from October 2020 to September 2021. A total of 377 CBCT scans samples were retrieved from the database by using the convenience sampling technique, out of which 123 CBCT scans fulfilled the inclusion criteria; these were all intact first permanent molars of both genders, with mature apex, and aged from 12–58 years. A total of 254 CBCT scans were excluded for various reasons such as permanent molars with root canal treatment, periapical infections, severe calcification or resorption, inaccurate

CBCT scans, compromised anatomy caused by physiological or pathological processes, full-coverage restorations, or metallic restorations.

Permission was obtained from the director of the dental complex to have patients' demographic details such as gender, age, and CBCT scans to evaluate the number of roots and root canal morphology of maxillary and mandibular first molars.

Root canal morphology was classified according to Vertucci's classification system [27] that categorized the canal configurations into eight types as shown in Figure 1.

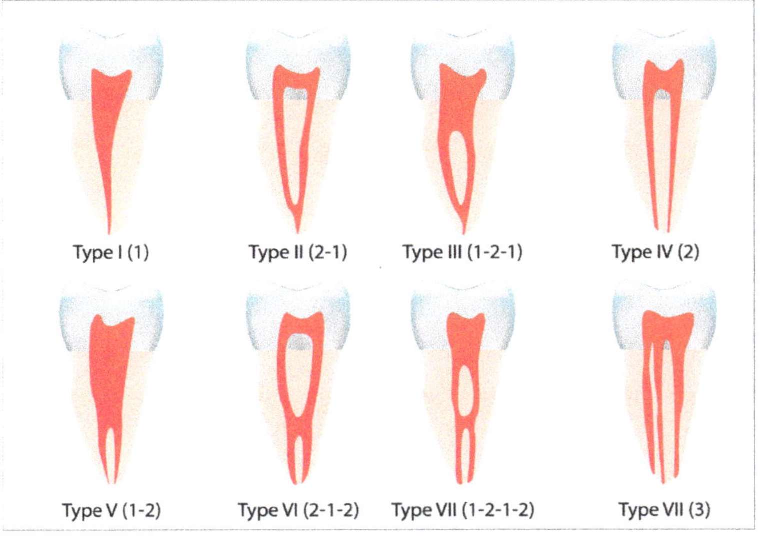

Figure 1. Schematic diagrams of Vertucci's Classification [27].

CBCT scans were captured with I-CAT Vision QTM (Imaging Sciences International, Hatfield, PA, USA. Version 1.9.3.14) 360-degree rotation scans with the field of view 130 with a voxel size of 0.25 mm at 0.250–0.400 Res, 120 kV, and 5 mA with exposure time 2–7 s. Inspection of images was done on a screen with an optimal view. Image brightness/contrast and magnification were adjusted to avoid mistakes and optimize visualization and interpretation. Gathering, interpretation, and recording of CBCT images were carried out by the principal investigator. BlueSkyPlan (Version 4.7.55, GmbH, Langenhagen, Germany) software was used to identify the number of roots and root canal configurations in sagittal, axial, and coronal views while following the checklist of Martins et al. [28].

Statistical Analysis

The collected data were analyzed using SPSS Version 21; IBM, Chicago, IL, USA. The number of roots, the number of canals and the configurations of all permanent first molars were documented as frequencies and percentages. Chi-square test was applied to evaluate the association of root canal morphology of mandibular and maxillary first molars with respect to gender. p-value < 0.05 was considered as statistical significant.

3. Results

A total of 123 CBCT images of the Saudi patients were assessed, out of which 59 (48.0%) were males and 64 (52.0%) were females; the mean age was 26.95 ± 10.65 years. All the patients 123 (100.0%) were Saudi nationals, as shown in Table 1.

Table 1. Demographic characteristics of participants (n = 123).

Variables		Mean ± SD n (%)
Age (years)		26.95 ± 10.65
Gender	Male	59 (48.0%)
	Female	64 (52.0%)
Nationality	Saudi	123 (100.0%)

Morphology of right maxillary first molar (FDI tooth # 16) revealed that three roots were prevalent in 111 (90.2%) cases while 12 (9.8%) cases had four roots. Three canals were prevalent in 97 (78.9%) cases while 26 (21.1%) cases had four canals. The majority of mesiobuccal root of right maxillary first molar had Type-I 107 (87.0%) of Vertucci classification followed by Type-IV 12 (9.8%), while only 4 (3.3%) patients had Type-II. Almost all palatal root 122 (99.2%) was Type-I and only 1 (0.8%) patient had additional Mesiopalatal canal MP (I). Morphology of left maxillary first molar (FDI tooth # 26) revealed that 111 (90.2%) cases had three roots while 12 (9.8%) cases had four roots. Three canals were prevalent in 94 (76.4%) cases while 29 (23.6%) cases had four canals. Most of the mesiobuccal root of left maxillary first molar was Type-I 104 (84.6%) followed by Type-IV 12 (9.8%), while only 7 (5.7%) patients had Type-II. No difference was found in palatal root finding of left maxillary and right maxillary molars. Distobuccal canal of all the bilateral maxillary first molars was Type-I. As far as other configuration of bilateral maxillary molars is concerned, it was observed that 10 (8.1%) had second mesiobuccal canal MB2 (I) and 1 (0.8%) had Disto-palatal DP (I), as shown in Table 2.

Table 2. Distribution of the morphology of the root canal according to Vertucci classification in maxillary first molars.

Variables			n (%)
Tooth # 16 (first molar right side)	mesio-buccal (MB)	I	107 (87.0%)
		II	4 (3.3%)
		III	0 (0%)
		IV	12 (9.8%)
	distobuccal (DB)	I	123 (100.0%)
	Palatal	I	122 (99.2%)
		Mesiopalatal MP (I)	1 (0.8%)
	other configuration	Second mesiobuccal canal MB2 (I)	10 (8.1%)
		Disto-palatal DP (I)	1 (0.8%)
		No	112 (91.1%)
	Number of Roots	3	111 (90.2%)
		4	12 (9.8%)
	Number of Canals	3	97 (78.9%)
		4	26 (21.1%)
Tooth # 26 (first molar left side)	mesio-buccal (MB)	I	104 (84.6%)
		II	7 (5.7%)
		IV	12 (9.8%)
	Disto buccal (DB)	I	123 (100.0%)
	Palatal	I	122 (99.2%)
		Mesiopalatal (I)	1 (0.8%)
	other configuration	Second mesiobuccal canal.MB2 (I)	10 (8.1%)
		Disto-palatal DP (I)	1 (0.8%)
		No	112 (91.1%)
	Number of Roots	3	111 (90.2%)
		4	12 (9.8%)
	Number of Canals	3	94 (76.4%)
		4	29 (23.6%)

Morphology of left mandibular first molar (FDI tooth # 36) revealed that 105 (85.4%) cases had three roots followed by four roots in 15 (12.2%) cases. On the other hand, most of the patients 90 (73.2%) had three canals while 31 (25.2%) had four canals. All the patients 123 (100.0%) of mesiobuccal root of left mandibular first molar had Type-I of Vertucci's classification. Mesiolingual canal of 122 (99.2%) patients had Type-I followed by Type-II in 1 (0.8%) case. Morphology of Distal canal showed that 91 (74.0%) were Type-I, 9 (7.3%) were Type-II, 2 (1.6%) were Type-III, 3 (2.4%) each in Type-IV and V and 15 (12.2%) cases showed additional Distobuccal (I) canal. As far as other configuration is concerned, it was observed that only 15 (12.2%) had Distolingual (I) canal. Morphology of right mandibular first molar (FDI tooth # 16) revealed that 105 (85.4%) cases had three roots followed by four roots in 16 (13.0%) cases and two roots present in 2 (1.6%) cases. On the other hand, most of the patients 91 (74.0%) had three canals while 31 (25.2%) had four canals followed by two canals in 1 (0.8%) case. All the patients 123 (100.0%) of mesiobuccal root of right mandibular first molar was Type-I of Vertucci's classification. Mesiolingual canal of 122 (99.2%) patients was Type-I followed by Type-II in 1 (0.8%) case. Morphology of the Distal canal showed that 91 (74.0%) were Type-I, 7 (5.7%) were Type-II, 2 (1.6%) were Type-III, 5 (4.1%) were Type-IV and 2 (1.6%) were Type-V and 16 (13.0%) cases showed additional distobuccal (I) canal. As far as other configuration is concerned, it was found that only 16 (13.0%) had Distolingual (I), as shown in Table 3.

A significant association was observed between gender and number of canals in maxillary right first molar. Females showed significantly higher prevalence of three-root canal configuration in maxillary first molars of the right side compared to males, while a majority of males had four canals ($p = 0.004$). In contrast, an insignificant association was found between gender and number of roots and other configuration of maxillary right first molar ($p > 0.05$). Concerning maxillary left first molar, a significant association was observed between gender and number of canals. Most females had three canals compared to males ($p = 0.001$). Additionally, an insignificant association was found between gender and number of roots and other configurations of maxillary left first molar ($p > 0.05$), as shown in Table 4.

Table 3. Distribution of the morphology of the root canal according to Vertucci classification in mandibular first molars.

	Variable		n (%)
Tooth # 36 (first molar left side)	mesio-buccal (MB)	I	123 (100.0%)
	Mesiolingual (ML)	I	122 (99.2%)
		II	1 (0.8%)
	Distal	I	91 (74.0%)
		II	9 (7.3%)
		III	2 (1.6%)
		IV	3 (2.4%)
		V	3 (2.4%)
	other configuration	Distobuccal (I)	15 (12.2%)
		Distolingual (I)	15 (12.2%)
		No	108 (87.8%)
	Number of Roots	1	1 (0.8%)
		2	2 (1.6%)
		3	105 (85.4%)
		4	15 (12.2%)
	Number of Canals	1	1 (0.8%)
		2	1 (0.8%)
		3	90 (73.2%)
		4	31 (25.2%)

Table 3. *Cont.*

Variable			n (%)
Tooth # 46 (first molar right side)	mesio-buccal (MB)	I	123 (100.0%)
	Mesiolingual (ML)	I	122 (99.2%)
		II	1 (0.8%)
	Distal	I	91 (74.0%)
		II	7 (5.7%)
		III	2 (1.6%)
		IV	5 (4.1%)
		V	2 (1.6%)
	other configuration	Distobuccal (I)	16 (13.0%)
		Distolingual (I)	16 (13.0%)
		No	107 (87.0%)
	Number of Roots	2	2 (1.6%)
		3	105 (85.4%)
		4	16 (13.0%)
	Number of Canals	2	1 (0.8%)
		3	91 (74.0%)
		4	31 (25.2%)

Table 4. Association of prevalence of the morphology of the root canal types in maxillary first molars with respect to gender.

Variable			Male Mean ± S.D n (%)	Female Mean ± S.D n (%)	*p*-Value
Tooth # 16 (first molar right side)	Age (years)		27.57 ± 11.32	26.37 ± 10.05	0.534
	Nationality	Saudi	59 (100.0%)	64 (100.0%)	-
	mesio-buccal (MB)	I	48 (81.4%)	59 (92.2$)	0.195
		II	3 (5.1%)	1 (1.6%)	
		IV	8 (13.6%)	4 (6.3%)	
	distobuccal (DB)	I	59 (100.0%)	64 (100.0%)	-
	Palatal	I	58 (98.3%)	64 (100.0%)	0.296
		Mesiopalatal MP (I)	1 (1.7%)	0 (0.0%)	
	other configuration	Second mesiobuccal canal. MB2 (I)	7 (11.9%)	3 (4.7%)	0.193
		Disto-palatal DP (I)	1 (1.7%)	0 (0.0%)	
		No	51 (86.4%)	61 (95.3%)	
	Number of Roots	3	51 (86.4%)	60 (93.8%)	0.172
		4	8 (13.6%)	4 (6.3%)	
	Number of Canals	3	40 (67.8%)	57 (89.1%)	0.004
		4	19 (32.2%)	7 (10.9%)	
Tooth # 26 (first molar left side)	mesio-buccal (MB)	I	45 (76.3%)	59 (92.2%)	0.050
		II	5 (8.5%)	2 (3.1%)	
		IV	9 (15.3%)	3 (4.7%)	
	distobuccal (DB)	I	59 (100.0%)	64 (100.0%)	-
	Palatal	I	58 (98.3%)	64 (100.0%)	0.296
		Mesiopalatal MP (I)	1 (1.7%)	0 (0.0%)	
	other configuration	Second mesiobuccal canal. MB2 (I)	7 (11.9%)	3 (4.7%)	0.193
		Disto-palatal DP (I)	1 (1.7%)	0 (0.0%)	

Table 4. *Cont.*

Variable		**Male Mean ± S.D n (%)**	**Female Mean ± S.D n (%)**	***p*-Value**
	NO	51 (86.4%)	61 (95.3%)	
Number of Roots	3	51 (86.4%)	60 (93.8%)	0.172
	4	8 (13.6%)	4 (6.3%)	
Number of Canals	3	37 (62.7%)	57 (89.1%)	0.001
	4	22 (37.3%)	7 (10.9%)	

On the other hand, there was an insignificant association observed between gender and number of canals, number of roots, and other configurations of mandibular left and right first molars ($p > 0.05$), as shown in Table 5.

Table 5. Association of prevalence of the morphology of the root canal types in mandibular first molars with respect to gender.

	Variable		**Male n (%)**	**Female n (%)**	***p*-Value**
Tooth #36 (first molar left side)	Mesio-buccal (MB)	I	59 (100.0%)	64 (100.0%)	-
	Mesiolingual (ML)	I	59 (100.0%)	63 (98.4%)	0.335
		II	0 (0.0%)	1 (1.6%)	
	Distal	I	41 (69.5%)	50 (78.1%)	0.449
		II	4(6.8%)	5 (7.8%)	
		III	1 (1.7%)	1 (1.6%)	
		IV	1 (1.7%)	2 (3.1%)	
		V	3 (5.1%)	0 (0.0%)	
	other configuration	Distobuccal (I)	9 (15.3%)	6 (9.4%)	0.320
		Distolingual (I)	9 (15.3%)	6 (9.4%)	
		No	50 (84.7%)	58 (90.6%)	
	Number of Roots	1	1 (1.7%)	0 (0.0%)	0.276
		2	0 (0.0%)	2 (3.1%)	
		3	49 (83.1%)	56 (87.5%)	
		4	9 (15.3%)	6 (9.4%)	
	Number of Canals	1	1 (1.7%)	0 (0.0%)	0.293
		2	0 (0.0%)	1 (1.6%)	
		3	40 (67.8%)	50 (78.1%)	
		4	18 (30.5%)	13 (20.3%)	
Tooth# 46 (first molar right side)	mesio-buccal (MB)	I	59 (100.0%)	64 (100.0%)	-
	mesiolingual (ML)	I	59 (100.0%)	63 (98.4%)	0.335
		II	0 (0.0%)	1 (1.6%)	
	Distal	I	40 (67.8%)	51 (79.7%)	0.178
		II	5 (8.5%)	2 (3.1%)	
		III	0 (0.0%)	2 (3.1%)	
		IV	2 (3.4%)	3 (4.7%)	
		V	2 (3.4%)	0 (0.0%)	
	other configuration	Distobuccal (I)	10 (16.9%)	6 (9.4%)	0.212
		Distolingual (I)	10 (16.9%)	6 (9.4%)	
		No	49 (83.1%)	58 (90.6%)	
	Number of Roots	2	1 (1.7%)	1 (1.6%)	0.456
		3	48 (81.4%)	57 (89.1%)	
		4	10 (16.9%)	6 (9.4%)	
	Number of Canals	2	1 (1.7%)		0.120
		3	39 (66.1%)	52 (81.3%)	
		4	19 (32.2%)	12 (18.8%)	

Initially, a panoramic image of patients was used for a general dental evaluation and select cases according to inclusion criteria as shown in Figure 2. An axial view of the maxillary arch was used to evaluate the number of roots and canals in maxillary molars as shown in Figure 3. Subsequently, the coronal view was used to evaluate the type of Vertucci's classification in the palatal root of maxillary first molar as shown in Figure 4.

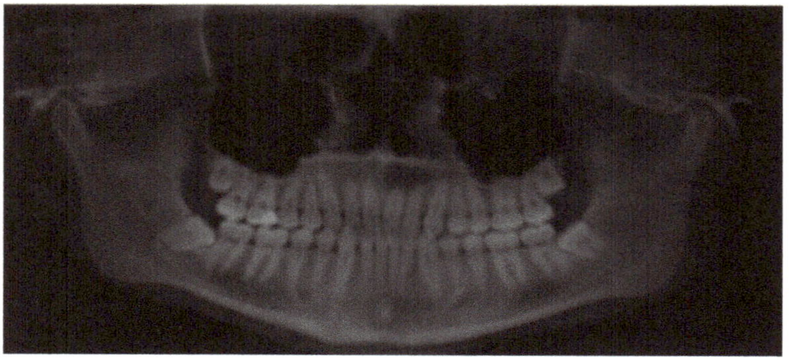

Figure 2. Panoramic view showing intact all permanent first molars.

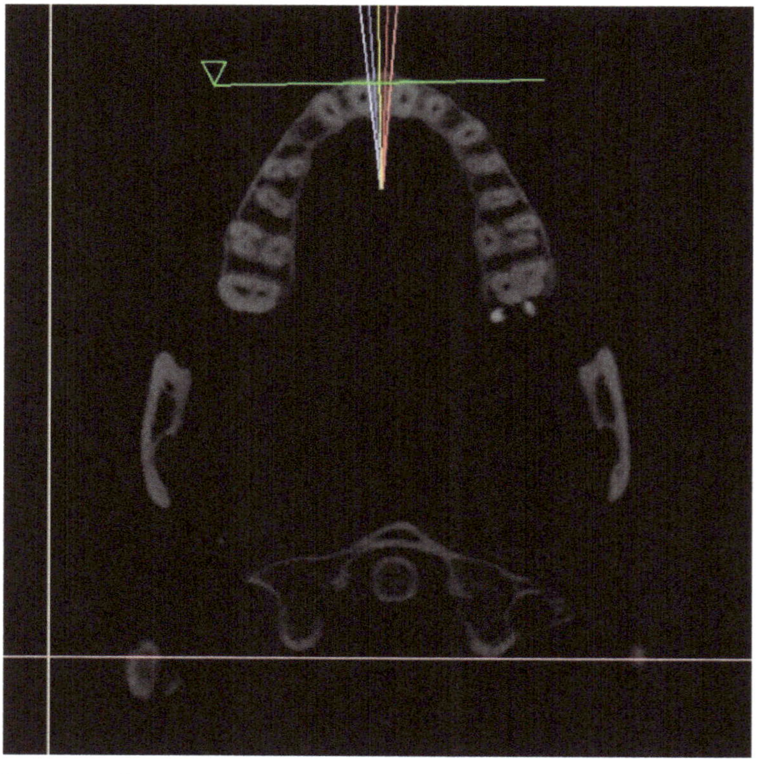

Figure 3. Axial view of maxillary arch showing number of roots and canals in maxillay molars.

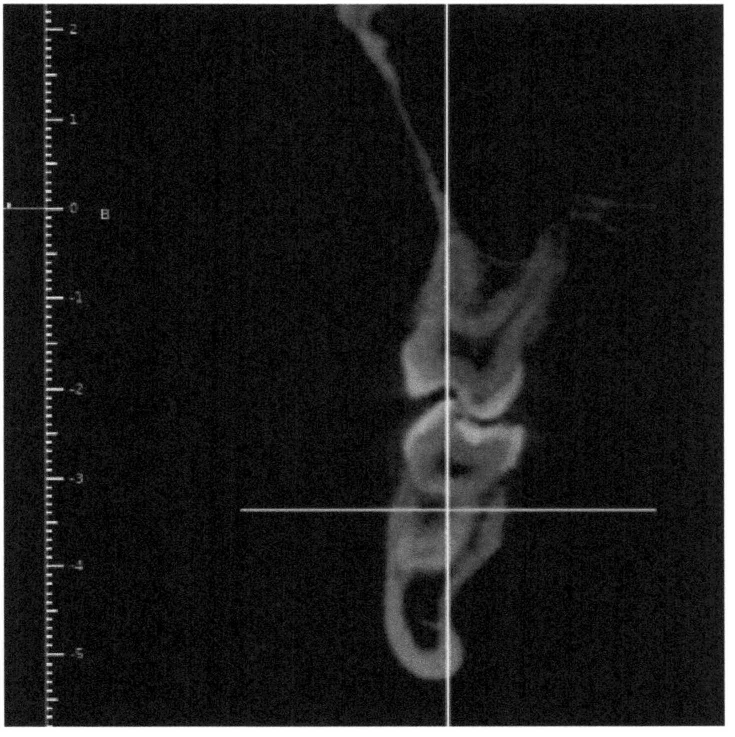

Figure 4. Coronal view of maxillary right molar (#16) showing Vertucci's Type-I canal configuration.

4. Discussion

It is imperative to ponder the complicated three-dimensional root canal morphology and probable variations to have successful endodontic treatment. A detailed theoretical interpretation, and hence an understanding of root canal morphology, can significantly diminish the problematic tasks encountered in access cavity preparation, cleaning and shaping, obturation, and final restoration of the root canal system [29].

The clinical efficiency of endodontic treatment procedures is dependent on a comprehensive knowledge of root structure and variance probability in root canal configuration, as undetected root canals lead to a treatment failure [30]. The present study demonstrated the root structure and root canal configuration of maxillary and mandibular first molars by using CBCT and its association with gender in the Saudi population.

Recently in clinical dental practice, the application of CBCT has gained admiration. With its non-invasive technique, CBCT supports dental practitioners in the diagnosis of endodontic problems along with a correct management plan. CBCT has been demonstrated as dependable and auspicious in identifying root canal structures in comparison with typical visual examination through physical tooth sectioning [31]. In 2015, the *American Association of Endodontists and American Academy of Oral and Maxillofacial Radiology Joint Position Statement* proposed that dental practitioners were recommended to apply CBCT merely while conventional dental radiography was unable to satisfactorily capture the images [32].

Interestingly, the accuracy of identifying additional canals is dependent on the voxel measurement and contrast resolution application. The present study scanned the maxillary and mandibular first molar teeth with voxel size 0.25 mm at 0.250–0.400 Res which gives an optimal view. This was endorsed by Bauman et al., who signified the resolution in the CBCT system that is $\leq$0.2 mm voxel sizes are optimum for the recognition of MBR canals [33]. Similarly, another research supported the CBCT system wherein all CBCT machines were fixed at 0.3 mm voxel size (14-bit grayscale) which gave optimal results [34].

This voxel measurement offered better diagnostic management and minimized the radiation dose; additionally, it looks suspicious that it had a great influence on the reliability of extra canal detection [33,35].

The present study showed that maxillary and mandibular first molars had three separate root canals, which were consistent with another research project wherein most of the first molars had three separate root canals (94%) [34]. These findings showed similarities with the former CBCT results in Saudi [19] and Brazilian populations [36].

The second mesiobuccal canal (MB2) is one of the most commonly undetected canals in maxillary molars that escapes the pulp chamber at a critical mesial inclination, and consequently bends distally making the task difficult for dental practitioners [37]. The present study showed that the prevalence of an MB2 in maxillary first molars was 10 (8.1%), which was not in accordance with other CBCT research wherein the prevalence of an MB2 was reported at 36.3% [38], <50% [39] and 73.8% [40]. Furthermore, our result is contrary to a Micro-CT based study [41] which showed that MB2 was present in 80% of the first maxillary molar. These differences in the results may be accredited to dissimilar sample sizes, ethnic groups, and approach variances. Previous studies showing the presence of MB2 canal in maxillary first molar in different populations is summarized in Table 6.

Table 6. Studies show in the presence of MB2 canal in maxillary first molar in different population.

Studies	Year	Population	CBCT Scans	Number of Canals in the Maxillary First Molar
Kim et al. [9]	2012	Korean	814	Additional canals were found in 63.59% of the mesiobuccal (MB) roots
Silva et al. [36]	2014	Brazilian	314	The prevalence of MB2 canal was 44.4%
Martin et al. [40]	2018	Indian	250	MB2 proportion in USA was 64.8%.
Al Mheiri et al. [42]	2020	Emirati	261	MB2 canal was found in 80.1% of all examined samples.
Martin et al. [40]	2018	Australian	250	50.8% samples had MB2 canal
Martin et al. [43]	2017	Caucasian	542	The mesiobuccal root of the maxillary first molars had two root canals in 71%
Heibert et al. [44]	2017	American	100	A review of CBCT volumes found the presence of an MB2 canal 69% of the time.
ABARCA et al. [45]	2015	Chilean	802	The presence of the MB2 canal in maxillary first was 32.5%.
Jing et al. [46]	2014	Chinese	630	30.9% maxillary molars had the additional canal in the mesio-buccal roots.
Naseri et al. [47]	2016	Irani	149	Additional canal (MB2) was detected in 86.6% of mesiobuccal roots

Besides MB2, the prevalence of second palatal canal in maxillary molars is rare. However, the present study identified the prevalence of second palatal canal 1 (0.8%) that was consistent with other research that observed the prevalence of a second palatal canal at 0.9% in maxillary first molars [38], and also in agreement with the further research by Ratanajirasut et al. [48] and Martins et al. [49] who revealed the existence of two palatal canals 1.7% of maxillary first molars in the Caucasian group.

Similarly, the present study showed that mandibular first molars of both sides had Type-I configuration, these findings showing inconsistency with findings reported in the studies by Pan et al. [38], Miloglu et al. [50], and Kim et al. [46] wherein most of the mandibular first molars had Type-IV configuration in the mesial root. These variations may be due to differences in sampling populations such as Malaysian, Turkish and Korean populations, respectively, selected in those research projects.

As far as the distal root is concerned, the present study revealed the prevalence of two distal canals in the distal root of mandibular first molars wherein the second distal canal in the distolingual position was found to be 15 (12.2%) of Type I configuration. These findings partly corroborated with the study by Martins et al. [49] that revealed a 19.5%

prevalence rate for a second distal canal in mandibular first molars. Conversely, one of the research projects conducted on the Sudanese population by Ahmed et al. [51] found a higher prevalence of 59% for two canals in distal roots of mandibular first molars. These variations may be due to differences in the sampling population.

Regarding the association of mesiobuccal root of maxillary molar teeth with gender, the present study revealed that mesiobuccal root had Vertucci Type-I that was more common in females, though there was a statistically insignificant difference in comparison with males ($p > 0.05$). These results corresponded strongly with the study conducted in North America by Guo et al. [47], who assessed maxillary first molars and established that Vertucci classification of Type-I was more commonly found in females than males even though there was a statistically insignificant difference between them. Additionally, further research by Betancourt et al. [52] in Chile and Jing et al. [53] in China, also reported that females had a significantly increased prevalence of single-root canal in the maxillary first molar. Remarkably, the present study contradicted the two studies by Altunsoy et al. [54] that were performed on a Turkish population and Naseri et al. [55] on an Iranian population, which supported that males had a higher prevalence of Vertucci Type-I configurations in mesial buccal roots of bilateral maxillary first molars although insignificant association was observed.

The present study concluded that the majority of cases in mandibular first permanent molars of both sides had 3 roots and three canals with insignificant association with gender ($p > 0.05$). These findings were in line with Deng et al.'s [56] research in the population of East Coast Malaysia.

The results of the present study must be seen under certain limitations. The data in the present study were acquired from a single center that maybe limited its methodology. Secondly, after following the exclusion criteria we ended up with 123 patients' CBCT images with a mean age of 26.95 ± 10.65 years, which is unlikely to represent the all-age group. Therefore, multicenter studies with wider age brackets are recommended for better representation of the population in the future. Additionally, to yield stronger conclusions it is preferable to perform this anatomical study over an extensive geographical range with racial variables. The present study evaluated the root canal morphology of permanent first molars in the Al Ahsa region population that used a voxel size of 0.25 mm and limits the study outcomes. Moreover, visualization of the morphology of root canals can be improved by using a high-resolution imaging modality such as Micro-CT [57,58]. CBCT is an operational, high-precision diagnostic tool for precise anatomical details. Nonetheless, high cost and radiation dose limit its clinical application. Consequently, better outcomes of endodontic treatment can be greatly developed by the acquaintance of clinicians with different root and canal morphological configurations.

5. Conclusions

This study concluded that the majority of maxillary and mandibular first molars had three roots and three canals with Type-I Vertucci's classification. In addition, gender was significantly associated with the number of canals in the maxillary molar, with females showing a greater tendency to have three canals than males. However, multicenter studies with a wider age bracket are recommended for better representation of the population in the future.

Author Contributions: Conceptualization, R.R.A., R.J., M.A.A.; methodology, R.J., M.A.A.; software, R.R.A., A.A.A., M.T.A., R.J.; validation, R.J., M.A.A., N.A.; formal analysis, R.J., M.A.A., N.A.; investigation, R.R.A., A.A.A., M.T.A., M.A.A., R.J.; resources, R.R.A., A.A.A., M.T.A., R.J.; data curation, R.J., M.A.A., N.A.; writing—original draft preparation, R.J., M.A.A.; writing—review and editing, M.A.A., R.J., N.A.; visualization, M.A.A., R.J.; supervision and project administration, R.J., M.A.A.; funding acquisition, R.R.A., R.J. All authors have read and agreed to the published version of the manuscript.

Funding: This work was supported by the Deanship of Scientific Research, Vice Presidency for Graduate Studies and Scientific Research, King Faisal University, Saudi Arabia (Project No. GRANT699).

Institutional Review Board Statement: The study was conducted in accordance with the Declaration of Helsinki, and approved by the Research Ethics Committee of Deanship of Scientific Research at King Faisal University (KFU-REC/2020-10-21).

Data Availability Statement: The data presented in this study are available on request from the corresponding author. The data are not publicly available due to privacy and ethical concern.

Acknowledgments: The authors are grateful to the Deanship of Scientific Research, Vice Presidency for Graduate Studies and Scientific Research, King Faisal University, Saudi Arabia for facilitating this project.

Conflicts of Interest: The authors declare no conflict of interest. The funders had no role in the design of the study; in the collection, analyses, or interpretation of data; in the writing of the manuscript, or in the decision to publish the results.

References

1. Tabassum, S.; Khan, F.R. Failure of endodontic treatment: The usual suspects. *Eur. J. Dent.* **2016**, *10*, 144–147. [CrossRef]
2. Karamifar, K.; Tondari, A.; Saghiri, M.A. Endodontic Periapical Lesion: An Overview on the Etiology, Diagnosis and Current Treatment Modalities. *Eur. Endod. J.* **2020**, *5*, 54–67. [CrossRef] [PubMed]
3. Ahmad, I.A.; Alenezi, M.A. Root and Root Canal Morphology of Maxillary First Premolars: A Literature Review and Clinical Considerations. *J. Endod.* **2016**, *42*, 861–872. [CrossRef] [PubMed]
4. Qiao, X.; Xu, T.; Chen, L.; Yang, D. Analysis of Root Canal Curvature and Root Canal Morphology of Maxillary Posterior Teeth in Guizhou, China. *Med. Sci. Monit.* **2021**, *27*, e928758. [CrossRef] [PubMed]
5. Baruwa, A.; Martins, J.; Meirinhos, J.; Pereira, B.; Gouveia, J.; Quaresma, S.; Monroe, A.; Ginjeira, A. The Influence of Missed Canals on the Prevalence of Periapical Lesions in Endodontically Treated Teeth: A Cross-sectional Study. *J. Endod.* **2020**, *46*, 34–39.e1. [CrossRef] [PubMed]
6. Pereira, B.; Martins, J.; Baruwa, A.; Meirinhos, J.; Gouveia, J.; Quaresma, S.; Monroe, A.; Ginjeira, A. Association between Endodontically Treated Maxillary and Mandibular Molars with Fused Roots and Periapical Lesions: A Cone-beam Computed Tomography Cross-sectional Study. *J. Endod.* **2020**, *46*, 771–777.e1. [CrossRef]
7. Vertucci, F.J. Root canal morphology and its relationship to endodontic procedure. *Endod. Topics* **2005**, *10*, 3–29. [CrossRef]
8. Hasan, M.; Khan, F.R. Determination of Frequency of the Second Mesiobuccal Canal in the Permanent Maxillary First Molar Teeth with Magnification Loupes (×3.5). *Int. J. Biomed. Sci.* **2014**, *10*, 201–207. [PubMed]
9. Kim, Y.; Lee, S.J.; Woo, J. Morphology of maxillary first and second molars analyzed by cone-beam computed tomography in a korean population: Variations in the number of roots and canals and the prevalence of fusion. *J. Endod.* **2012**, *38*, 1063–1068. [CrossRef]
10. Abd-Latib, A.H.; Nordin, N.F.; Alkadhim, A.H. CBCT diagnostic application in detection of mesiobuccal canal in maxillary molars and distolingual canal in mandibular molars: A descriptive study. *J. Dent. Oral Health* **2015**, *1*, 1–3.
11. Studebaker, B.; Hollender, L.; Mancl, L.; Johnson, J.D.; Paranjpe, A. The Prevalence of Second Mesiobuccal Canals Located in Maxillary Molars with the Aid of Cone-beam Computed Tomography. *J. Endod.* **2018**, *44*, 565–570. [CrossRef]
12. AL-Alawi, H.; Al-Nazhan, S.; Al-Maflehi, N.; Aldosimani, M.A.; Zahid, M.N.; Shihabi, G.N. The prevalence of radix molaris in the mandibular first molars of a Saudi subpopulation based on cone-beam computed tomography. *Restor. Dent. Endod.* **2020**, *45*, e1. [CrossRef] [PubMed]
13. Nur, B.G.; Ok, E.; Altunsoy, M.; Aglarci, O.S.; Colak, M.; Gungor, E. Evaluation of the root and canal morphology of mandibular permanent molars in a south-eastern Turkish population using cone-beam computed tomography. *Eur. J. Dent.* **2014**, *8*, 154–159. [CrossRef] [PubMed]
14. Wang, Y.; Zheng, Q.H.; Zhou, X.D.; Tang, L.; Wang, Q.; Zheng, G.N.; Huang, D.M. Evaluation of the root and canal morphology of mandibular first permanent molars in a western Chinese population by cone-beam computed tomography. *J. Endod.* **2010**, *36*, 1786–1789. [CrossRef] [PubMed]
15. Park, J.B.; Kim, N.; Park, S.; Kim, Y.; Ko, Y. Evaluation of root anatomy of permanent mandibular premolars and molars in a Korean population with cone-beam computed tomography. *Eur. J. Dent.* **2013**, *7*, 94–101.
16. Shukla, S.; Chug, A.; Afrashtehfar, K.I. Role of Cone Beam Computed Tomography in Diagnosis and Treatment Planning in Dentistry: An Update. *J. Int. Soc. Prev. Community Dent.* **2017**, *7*, S125–S136.
17. Venkatesh, E.; Elluru, S.V. Cone beam computed tomography: Basics and applications in dentistry. *J. Istanb. Univ. Fac. Dent.* **2017**, *51*, S102–S121. [CrossRef]
18. Witherspoon, D.E.; Small, J.C.; Regan, J.D. Missed canal systems are the most likely basis for endodontic retreatment of molars. *Tex. Dent. J.* **2013**, *130*, 127–139.
19. Al-Fouzan, K.S.; Ounis, H.F.; Merdad, K.; Al-Hezaimi, K. Prevalence of canal systems in the mesio-buccal roots of maxillary first and second molars in Saudi Arabian population. *Aust. Endod. J.* **2013**, *39*, 98–101. [CrossRef]

20. Alrahabi, M.; Sohail-Zafar, M. Evaluation of root canal morphology of maxillary molars using cone beam computed tomography. *Pak. J. Med. Sci.* **2015**, *31*, 426–430. [CrossRef]
21. Blinov, V.S.; Kartashov, M.V.; Zholudev, S.E.; Zornikova, O.S. Estimation of the cone-beam computed tomography in diagnostics of the molar root system anatomy of the mandible and maxilla. *Radiol. Pract.* **2016**, *59*, 6–15.
22. Filpo-Perez, C.; Bramante, C.M.; Villas-Boas, M.H.; Húngaro-Duarte, M.A.; Versiani, M.A.; Ordinola-Zapata, R. Micro-computed tomographic analysis of the root canal morphology of the distal root of mandibular first molar. *J. Endod.* **2015**, *41*, 231–236. [CrossRef] [PubMed]
23. Dinakar, C.; Shetty, U.A.; Salian, V.V.; Shetty, P. Root canal morphology of maxillary first premolars using the clearing technique in a south Indian population: An in vitro study. *Int. J. Appl. Basic Med. Res.* **2018**, *8*, 143–147. [CrossRef] [PubMed]
24. Patel, S.; Durack, C.; Abella, F.; Shemesh, H.; Roig, M.; Lemberg, K. Cone beam computed tomography in endodontics–a review. *Int. Endod. J.* **2015**, *48*, 3–15. [CrossRef] [PubMed]
25. Neelakantan, P.; Subbarao, C.; Subbarao, C.V. Comparative evaluation of modified canal staining and clearing technique, cone-beam computed tomography, peripheral quantitative computed tomography, spiral computed tomography, and plain and contrast medium–enhanced digital radiography in studying root canal morphology. *J. Endod.* **2010**, *36*, 1547–1551.
26. Zheng, Q.H.; Wang, Y.; Zhou, X.D.; Wang, Q.; Zheng, G.N.; Huang, D.M. A cone-beam computed tomography study of maxillary first permanent molar root and canal morphology in a Chinese population. *J. Endod.* **2010**, *36*, 1480–1484. [CrossRef]
27. Vertucci, F.J. Root canal anatomy of the human permanent teeth. *Oral Surg. Oral Med. Oral Pathol.* **1984**, *58*, 589–599. [CrossRef]
28. Martins, J.; Kishen, A.; Marques, D.; Nogueira Leal Silva, E.; Caramês, J.; Mata, A.; Versiani, M. Preferred Reporting Items for Epidemiologic Cross-sectional Studies on Root and Root Canal Anatomy Using Cone-beam Computed Tomographic Technology: A Systematized Assessment. *J. Endod.* **2020**, *46*, 915–935. [CrossRef]
29. Domark, J.D.; Hatton, J.F.; Benison, R.P.; Hildebolt, C.F. An ex vivo comparison of digital radiography and cone-beam and micro computed tomography in the detection of the number of canals in the mesiobuccal roots of maxillary molars. *J. Endod.* **2013**, *39*, 901–905. [CrossRef]
30. Al-Zubaidi, S.M.; Almansour, M.I.; Al-Mansour, N.N.; Alshammari, A.S.; Alshammari, A.F.; Altamimi, Y.S.; Madfa, A.A. Assessment of root morphology and canal configuration of maxillary premolars in a Saudi subpopulation: A cone-beam computed tomographic study. *BMC Oral Health* **2021**, *21*, 397. [CrossRef]
31. Khanna, A.B. Applications of cone beam computed tomography in endodontics. *Evid.-Based Endod.* **2020**, *5*, 1. [CrossRef]
32. American Association of Endodontics and American Academy of Oral and Maxillofacial Radiology. AAE and AAOMR joint position statement: Use of cone beam computed tomography in endodontics 2015 update. *J. Endod.* **2015**, *41*, 1393–1396. [CrossRef] [PubMed]
33. Bauman, R.; Scarfe, W.; Clark, S.; Morelli, J.; Scheetz, J.; Farman, A. Ex vivo detection of mesiobuccal canals in maxillary molars using CBCT at four different isotropic voxel dimensions. *Int. Endod. J.* **2011**, *44*, 752–758. [CrossRef] [PubMed]
34. Al-Shehri, S.; Al-Nazhan, S.; Shoukry, S.; Al-Shwaimi, E.; Al-Sadhan, R.; Al-Shemmery, B. Root and canal configuration of the maxillary first molar in a Saudi subpopulation: A cone-beam computed tomography study. *Saudi. Endod. J.* **2017**, *7*, 69–76.
35. Vizzotto, M.B.; Silveira, P.F.; Arús, N.A.; Montagner, F.; Gomes, B.P.; da Silveira, H.E. CBCT for the assessment of second mesiobuccal (MB2) canals in maxillary molar teeth: Effect of voxel size and presence of root filling. *Int. Endod. J.* **2013**, *46*, 870–876. [CrossRef]
36. Silva, E.J.; Nejaim, Y.; Silva, A.I.; Haiter-Neto, F.; Zaia, A.A.; Cohenca, N. Evaluation of root canal configuration of maxillary molars in a Brazilian population using cone-beam computed tomographic imaging: An in vivo study. *J. Endod.* **2014**, *40*, 173–176. [CrossRef]
37. Görduysus, M.O.; Görduysus, M.; Friedman, S. Operating microscope improves negotiation of second mesiobuccal canals in maxillary molars. *J. Endod.* **2001**, *27*, 683–686. [CrossRef]
38. Pan, J.Y.Y.; Parolia, A.; Chuah, S.R.; Bhatia, S.; Mutalik, S.; Pau, A. Root canal morphology of permanent teeth in a Malaysian subpopulation using cone-beam computed tomography. *BMC Oral Health.* **2019**, *19*, 14. [CrossRef]
39. Aktan, A.M.; Yildirim, C.; Culha, E.; Demir, E.; Ertugrul-Ciftci, M. Detection of Second Mesiobuccal Canals in Maxillary First Molars Using a New Angle of Cone Beam Computed Tomography. *Iran. J. Radiol.* **2016**, *13*, e31155. [CrossRef]
40. Martins, J.N.R.; Alkhawas, M.A.M.; Altaki, Z.; Bellardini, G.; Berti, L.; Boveda, C.; Chaniotis, A.; Flynn, D.; Gonzalez, J.A.; Kottoor, J.; et al. Worldwide Analyses of Maxillary First Molar Second Mesiobuccal Prevalence: A Multicenter Cone-beam Computed Tomographic Study. *J. Endod.* **2018**, *44*, 1641–1649.e1. [CrossRef]
41. Alfouzan, K.; Alfadley, A.; Alkadi, L.; Alhezam, A.; Jamleh, A. Detecting the Second Mesiobuccal Canal in Maxillary Molars in a Saudi Arabian Population: A Micro-CT Study. *Scanning* **2019**, *2019*, 9568307. [CrossRef] [PubMed]
42. Al Mheiri, E.; Chaudhry, J.; Abdo, S.; El Abed, R.; Khamis, A.H.; Jamal, M. Evaluation of root and canal morphology of maxillary permanent first molars in an Emirati population; a cone-beam computed tomography study. *BMC Oral Health* **2020**, *20*, 274. [CrossRef] [PubMed]
43. Martins, J.N.; Marques, D.; Mata, A.; Caramês, J. Root and root canal morphology of the permanent dentition in a Caucasian population: A cone-beam computed tomography study. *Int. Endod. J.* **2017**, *50*, 1013–1026. [CrossRef] [PubMed]
44. Hiebert, B.M.; Abramovitch, K.; Rice, D.; Torabinejad, M. Prevalence of second mesiobuccal canals in maxillary first molars detected using cone-beam computed tomography, direct occlusal access, and coronal plane grinding. *J. Endod.* **2017**, *43*, 1711–1715. [CrossRef]

45. Abarca, J.; Gómez, B.; Zaror, C.; Monardes, H.; Bustos, L.; Cantin, M. Assessment of mesial root morphology and frequency of MB2 canals in maxillary molars using cone beam computed tomography. *Int. J. Morphol.* **2015**, *33*, 1333–1337. [CrossRef]
46. Kim, S.Y.; Kim, B.S.; Woo, J.; Kim, Y. Morphology of mandibular first molars analyzed by cone-beam computed tomography in a Korean population: Variations in the number of roots and canals. *J. Endod.* **2013**, *39*, 1516–1521. [CrossRef]
47. Guo, J.; Vahidnia, A.; Sedghizadeh, P.; Enciso, R. Evaluation of root and canal morphology of maxillary permanent first molars in a North American population by cone-beam computed tomography. *J. Endod.* **2014**, *40*, 635–639. [CrossRef]
48. Ratanajirasut, R.; Panichuttra, A.; Panmekiate, S. A cone-beam computed tomographic study of root and canal morphology of maxillary first and second permanent molars in a Thai population. *J. Endod.* **2018**, *44*, 56–61. [CrossRef]
49. Martins, J.N.R.; Gu, Y.; Marques, D.; Francisco, H.; Caramês, J. Differences on the root and root canal morphologies between Asian and Caucasian ethnic groups analyzed by cone beam computed tomography. *J. Endod.* **2018**, *44*, 1096–1104. [CrossRef] [PubMed]
50. Miloglu, O.; Arslan, H.; Barutcigil, C.; Cantekin, K. Evaluating root and canal configuration of mandibular first molars with cone beam computed tomography in a Turkish population. *J. Dent. Sci.* **2013**, *8*, 80–86. [CrossRef]
51. Ahmed, H.A.; Abu-bakr, N.H.; Yahia, N.A.; Ibrahim, Y.E. Root and canal morphology of permanent mandibular molars in a Sudanese population. *Int. Endod. J.* **2007**, *40*, 766–771. [CrossRef] [PubMed]
52. Betancourt, P.; Navarro, P.; Muñoz, G.; Fuentes, R. Prevalence and location of the secondary mesiobuccal canal in 1,100 maxillary molars using cone beam computed tomography. *BMC Med. Imaging.* **2016**, *16*, 66. [CrossRef] [PubMed]
53. Jing, Y.; Ye, X.; Liu, D.; Zhang, Z.; Ma, X. Cone-beam computed tomography was used for study of root and canal morphology of first and second molars. *Beijing Da Xue Xue Bao. Yi Xue Ban J. Peking Univ. Health Sci.* **2014**, *46*, 958–962.
54. Altunsoy, M.; Ok, E.; Nur, B.; Aglarci, O.; Gungor, E.; Colak, M. Root canal morphology analysis of maxillary permanent first and second molars in a southeastern Turkish population using cone-beam computed tomography. *J. Dent. Sci.* **2015**, *10*, 401–407. [CrossRef]
55. Naseri, M.; Safi, Y.; Akbarzadeh-Baghban, A.; Khayat, A.; Eftekhar, L. Survey of Anatomy and Root Canal Morphology of Maxillary First Molars Regarding Age and Gender in an Iranian Population Using Cone-Beam Computed Tomography. *Iran. Endod. J.* **2016**, *11*, 298–303. [PubMed]
56. Deng, P.U.; Halim, M.S.; Masudi, S.M.; Al-Shehadat, S.; Ahmad, B. Cone-beam computed tomography analysis on root and canal morphology of mandibular first permanent molar among multiracial population in East Coast Malaysian population. *Eur. J. Dent.* **2018**, *12*, 410–416. [CrossRef] [PubMed]
57. Wolf, T.G.; Paqué, F.; Zeller, M.; Willershausen, B.; Briseño-Marroquín, B. Root Canal Morphology and Configuration of 118 Mandibular First Molars by Means of Micro-Computed Tomography: An Ex Vivo Study. *J Endod.* **2016**, *42*, 610–614. [CrossRef]
58. Briseño-Marroquín, B.; Paqué, F.; Maier, K.; Willershausen, B.; Wolf, T.G. Root Canal Morphology and Configuration of 179 Maxillary First Molars by Means of Micro-computed Tomography: An Ex Vivo Study. *J Endod.* **2015**, *41*, 2008–2013. [CrossRef]

diagnostics

MDPI

Review

The Use of CBCT in Evaluating the Health and Pathology of the Maxillary Sinus

Andy Wai Kan Yeung [1], Kuo Feng Hung [2], Dion Tik Shun Li [2] and Yiu Yan Leung [2,*]

[1] Oral and Maxillofacial Radiology, Applied Oral Sciences and Community Dental Care, Faculty of Dentistry, The University of Hong Kong, Hong Kong SAR, China
[2] Oral and Maxillofacial Surgery, Faculty of Dentistry, The University of Hong Kong, Hong Kong SAR, China
* Correspondence: mikeyyleung@hku.hk

Abstract: The use of cone-beam computed tomography (CBCT) has been increasing in dental practice. This narrative review summarized the relevance and utilizations of CBCT to visualize anatomical structures of the maxillary sinus and common pathologies found in the maxillary sinus. The detection/visualization rate, the location and the morphometric characteristics were described. For sinus anatomy, the reviewed features included the posterior superior alveolar artery, sinus pneumatization, sinus hypoplasia, sinus septa, and primary and accessory sinus ostia. For pathology, the following items were reviewed: membrane thickening associated with periapical lesions/periodontal lesions, mucous retention cyst, and antrolith. The visualization and assessment of the maxillary sinus is very important prior to procedures that take place in close proximity with the sinus floor, such as tooth extraction, implant insertion, and sinus floor elevation. Some sinus pathologies may be associated with odontogenic lesions, such as periapical diseases and periodontal bone loss.

Keywords: cone beam computed tomography; CBCT; maxillary sinus; Schneiderian membrane; health; pathology; sinus floor elevation

1. Introduction

The maxillary sinuses are a pair of large air-filled cavities located superior to the posterior part of the dentoalveolar region of the maxilla. The maxillary sinus has the shape of a pyramid and is the largest among the four paranasal sinuses. It drains into the middle meatus of the nasal cavity. It has three recesses, the alveolar process, the zygomatic recess, and the infraorbital recess. Due to the proximity of the sinus floor with the alveolar ridge, the maxillary sinus is of high relevance to multiple dental procedures, ranging from tooth extraction to implant insertion. When the sinus condition should be considered during diagnosis and treatment planning, the cone beam computed tomography (CBCT) is the optimal choice among the common imaging modalities, as it allows a 3D visualization of the structure either entirely or partially, and without the limitation of superimposition with other structures as with 2D imaging. It was reported that 10–14% of the population in Europe and the United States suffered from chronic sinusitis, which could be rhinosinusal or odontogenic [1]. Subsequently, pathologies of the paranasal sinuses were common incidental findings from CBCT imaging [2]. For example, panoramic radiography could not accurately demonstrate root proximity with the sinus floor when there was root contact with the sinus floor on the buccal or palatal side [3]. In these circumstances, panoramic radiography tended to overestimate the extent of root protrusion into the sinus [4], and could make the root appear to be in the sinus [5]. Similarly, panoramic radiography showed inferior performance in detecting sinus membrane thickening [6], sinus septum [7], or oroantral communication after tooth extraction [8]. On the other hand, anatomical variations of the maxillary sinus could sometimes "false positively" presented as apparent odontogenic lesions such as radicular cysts associated with maxillary teeth on a panoramic radiograph, which required further evaluation by CBCT [9].

Dental CBCT machines were developed and commercialized near the end of the 1990s and since then they have been heavily used in dental implant research to assess the condition of the maxillary sinus [10,11]. In fact, the European Academy of Dentomaxillofacial Radiology (EADMFR) advocated a minimum level and core content for training dentists who were involved in CBCT imaging and interpretation for general dentists [12]. In Level 1, a general dentist should be able to use CBCT machines, analyse normal anatomical structures of the teeth, jaws and facial skeleton in CBCT images, and recognize both anatomy and disease of the teeth and supporting structures in CBCT images [12]. In Level 2, a general dentist should be able to differentiate between findings indicating normal anatomical structures from those of diseased teeth, jaws and facial skeleton [12]. Therefore, the correct interpretation of the status of the maxillary sinus is one important aspect in reading CBCT images, as the sinus is frequently in close proximity of the root apices of the maxillary posterior teeth.

In clinical practice, one of the most frequent indications for dental CBCT imaging was the dimensional and health assessment of the alveolar ridge and maxillary sinus for implant planning and sinus lift procedures [13], including the assessment of the bone graft volume required [14]. Indeed, several authorities have advocated the use of CBCT for pre-operative evaluation of the implant planning sites [15–17]. Besides implant planning, evaluating the health status of the maxillary sinuses during the diagnostic and treatment planning procedures has also been suggested in other scenarios, such as orthodontics [18], pre-operative assessment of teeth undergoing apical surgery [19], and evaluation of cystic and neoplastic lesions in the maxillary region especially if the posterior region was involved [20].

As mentioned above, a CBCT scan produces a 3D image volume, and hence its radiation dose is usually higher than a plain radiograph such as a panoramic or a periapical radiograph. Some clinicians may thus minimize the use of CBCT and subsequently be unfamiliar with the advantages of this modality over plain radiography in evaluating the maxillary sinus. With the versatility of a CBCT machine, multiple parameters ranging from the spatial resolution, peak voltage to the number of projections can be adjusted to optimize the radiation dose emitted, such that the principle of "as low as reasonably achievable" (ALARA) has gone through a long history of evolution [21], with some expert opinions that advocated to rename it to "as low as diagnostically acceptable" (ALADA) [22] and, more recently, "as low as diagnostically acceptable being indication-oriented and patient-specific" (ALADAIP) [23]. One quality assurance measure to optimize the radiation dose is to establish institutional or national dose reference levels (DRLs) for each indication of CBCT examinations. For instance, it was suggested that the DRL for a CBCT examination to evaluate maxillary sinus pathology could be in the range of 520–1150 mGy $\times$ cm^2 [24]. Another measure is to enhance user training to minimize the chance of a retake due to inadequate diagnostic value of the original scan. It was recently reported that CBCT retake rate was approximately 2.8% across studies [25], and that inadequate visualization of the maxillary sinus was one of the commonest reasons for a retake [26].

The anatomical variants of the maxillary sinus are mainly sinus septations, presence of accessory sinus ostium, and sinus hypoplasia, among the others [27]. Meanwhile, its pathologies can generally be classified into inflammatory, iatrogenic, traumatic, neoplastic, odontogenic, congenital and bone-related [28]. This narrative review aimed to provide an overview of the findings from published CBCT studies that evaluated the anatomy and pathology of the maxillary sinus.

2. Anatomy

2.1. Posterior Superior Alveolar Artery (PSAA) and Lateral Wall Thickness

The PSAA is a branch of the maxillary artery that runs along and supplies the lateral wall of the maxillary sinus and the overlying Schneiderian membrane (Figure 1). It should be carefully considered during sinus grafting procedures as there may be a potential risk of profound bleeding [29]. Severe bleeding after damaging PSAA during sinus floor elevation with transcrestal technique has been documented [30]. The detection/visualization rate of

PSAA on CBCT scans ranged from around 48.6 to 91.6% [31–36]. PSAA could be mostly found below the sinus membrane (13–63.8%) or intraosseous (28.5–71.1%), but less frequent at the outer cortex of the lateral wall of the sinus (5.2–9.9%) [31–36]. The apparent absence of PSAA in some CBCT scans could be due to its small size or lying immediately on either side of the lateral wall of the sinus without forming bone indentation [36]. For a meta-analysis on the prevalence of PSAA in a pooled collection of CBCT and CT studies, readers should refer to [37].

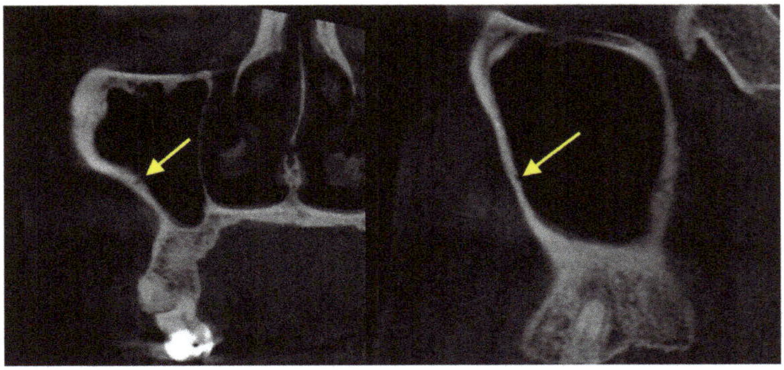

Figure 1. Posterior superior alveolar artery shown in CBCT.

Meanwhile, the lateral wall thickness of the maxillary sinus might be critically assessed by CBCT imaging during lateral sinus elevation procedures. A retrospective study of 209 patients with CBCT scans found that the overall mean lateral wall thickness was 1.6 ± 0.8 mm at both 4 mm and 6 mm apical (superior) to the sinus floor [38]. However, cases with membrane perforation during operation had a mean lateral wall thickness of 2.4 ± 0.6 mm at both 4 mm and 6 mm apical to the sinus floor, compared to 1.2 ± 0.4 mm for the non-perforation cases [38]. The lateral wall of the maxillary sinus was also found to be thicker in partial edentulism cases (1.3 ± 0.3 mm) compared to complete edentulism cases (1.0 ± 0.3 mm), and positively correlated with residual ridge height [39]. Considering the mesiodistal direction, the lateral wall thickness at 30–40 mm inferior to the orbital floor showed a gradual reduction from the canine region towards the second molar region [40]. There was a positive correlation between the diameter of PSAA and the thickness of the lateral wall of the maxillary sinus [41].

2.2. *Pneumatization*

Maxillary sinus pneumatization does not seem to have a precise definition. In general, it refers to the maxillary sinus extension into a particular anatomical structure, such as the alveolar ridge, maxillary tuberosity, and palate [42]. For instance, alveolar pneumatization was considered present if the maxillary sinus floor was coronal to the apex of one of the roots of the posterior teeth [43]. Its overall prevalence from CBCT studies ranged from 23.5% to 83.2% [42,43]. It was more common among patients aged between 18 and 34 years (66.4%), followed by those aged between 35–59 years (36.8%) and those aged 60 years or above (22.3%) [44]. It was believed that the alveolar pneumatization was the most common variant, involved in as many as 100% of patients with sinus pneumatization, followed by the palate/palatal process (23.6%), maxillary tuberosity (22%), and anterior region (5.2%) [42]. Alveolar pneumatization tended to be most severe between the first and second molars (13.8–14.0 mm), followed by between the second and third molars (13.22 mm) and between the second premolar and first molar (9.1–9.2 mm) [45]. Similarly, localized sinus pneumatization following tooth loss was more likely to occur at the first molar (37.9%), compared to the second molar (12.1%) [43]. After minimally traumatic molar extraction, alveolar ridge preservation with synthetic nanohydroxyapatite was found to associate with

0.7 mm sinus pneumatization, slightly smaller than the 1.0 mm from unassisted socket healing [46]. The difference was statistically insignificant [46]. For palatal pneumatization, most of them (>99%) did not extend medially to exceed one-half of the width of the nasal floor [47].

2.3. Hypoplasia

In contrast to sinus pneumatization, sinus hypoplasia leads to reduced sinus cavity volume. At first glance, this seems to be a favourable condition given the ample distance between the dentoalveolar region and the sinus floor. However, the presence of sinus hypoplasia in CBCT images was found to significantly increase the prevalence of sinus mucosal thickening and blocked ostium (68.3% vs. 25.6%) [48]. The prevalence of sinus hypoplasia was reported to be around 0.2–50% [42,48,49]. Most of the cases belonged to Type I (69.5%; mild hypoplasia, normal uncinate process, and patent infundibular tract) or Type II (25.6%; moderate hypoplasia, hypoplastic uncinate process, and ill-defined or absent infundibular tract). Type III accounted for a minority (4.9%; severe sinus hypoplasia and absence of uncinate process) [48]. In rare circumstances, aplasia might be found from CBCT imaging as an incidental finding [50]. Apart from sinus health, sinus hypoplasia did not seem to affect the health or functions of dentoalveolar structures, such as canting of the maxillary occlusal plane, open bite, or mandibular asymmetry [51].

2.4. Sinus Augmentation

In implant cases where the severely resorbed alveolar bone ridge was unable to accommodate an implant, sinus augmentation procedure should be performed to increase the amount of bone inferior to the maxillary sinus floor. Recent CBCT studies found that such bone graft volume decreased by an average of 25% after 4.7–6 months of healing [52,53]. From 6 months after grafting until 3 years after grafting, the graft volume could be reduced by an average of 27.4–39.3% [53,54]. However, one CBCT study found no such significant reduction in the graft volume 4–7 months after the surgery [55]. Apart from bone volume, the bone mineral density is also an important factor for successful implantation. The gray level measured at the implant sites in CBCT images was found to have a good correlation to the actual mineralized material content computed by microradiography of the bone core biopsies taken at the implant sites [56]. Additionally, the gray level of sites grated with bovine bone materials remained stable at 4–7 months of follow-up [55].

2.5. Septa

The presence of sinus septa at the sinus floor and lateral wall of the sinus may hinder sinus lift procedures (Figure 2). The prevalence of sinus septa was around 27.1–59.7% [42,57–60]. Septa could be orientated in a coronal direction (61.8–79.2%), axial direction (4.9–22.3%) or sagittal directions (3.6–24.5%) [57–59,61]. As many as 4 septa within one sinus have been reported [57,58]. In the caudocranial direction, septa was most prevalent in the sinus floor (58.6%), followed by roof (33.1%), anterior wall (6.7%), posterior wall (1.2%), and lateral/medial wall (0.4%) [57]. In the anteroposterior direction, septa was most prevalent in the region of the 1st and 2nd molars (37.2–69.1%), followed by the region of the third molar (18.6–33.0%) and the region of the canines and premolars (12.2–29.8%) [59,60].

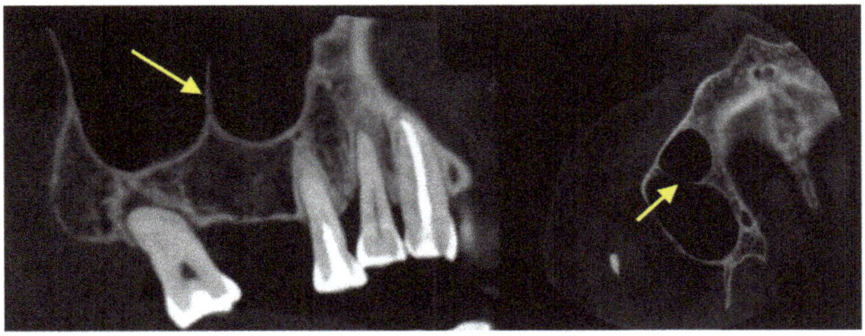

Figure 2. Nasal septum on the sinus floor.

2.6. Primary and Accessory Ostia

The sinus cavity is drained into the nasal cavity by mucociliary clearance system through the (primary) sinus ostium (Figure 3). Drainage is severed if the ostium is blocked. Ostium patency in CBCT images was found to be around 87.0–94.0% [62–64]. It is located above the attachment of the inferior turbinate, and most of the time it was located in the middle third (76.1%) of the turbinate or the anterior third (23.7%) [64]. Most sinus ostia were reported to be slit shaped (71.1%), followed by ovoloid (22.3%) and round (6.6%) [64]. Obstruction was significantly more likely to occur if the sinus had sinusitis or >10 mm membrane thickening [62,64]. Immediately after sinus floor elevation, it was estimated that obstruction occurred for up to 30% of the sinus ostia, which were mostly resolved at 7.5-month follow-up [63].

Meanwhile, the prevalence of accessory ostium was 35.5–56.7% [64–67]. Contrast to primary ostium, the accessory ostium was usually ovaloid (48.4%) or round (39.0%) instead of slit shaped (12.6%) [65]. The accessory ostium, if present, was on average 19.9 $\pm$ 1.7 mm from the most inferior point of the sinus floor [67]. The presence of sinusitis or mucosal thickening and accessory ostium were associated [66,67].

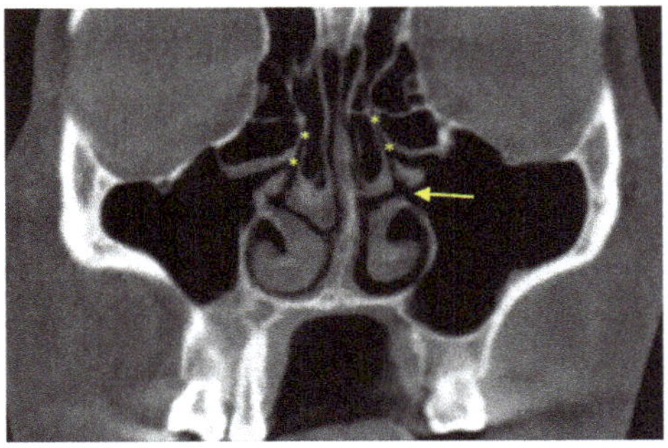

Figure 3. Primary ostium (asterisk) in both maxillary sinuses and accessory ostium (arrow) in the left maxillary sinus.

3. Pathology

3.1. Membrane Thickening Associated with Periapical Lesions

Sinus membrane thickening associated with an endodontically involved tooth was common (Figure 4). It has been reported by numerous studies [68–71]. In one study, the sinus membrane was, on average, 2.56–2.74 mm thick in cases with associated teeth having apical pathology, which was significantly thicker than the healthy controls (1.18–1.21 mm) [70]. In another study, the prevalence of membrane thickening was reported to be 41.5% for patients with no associated teeth with apical periodontitis, but increased to around 70% for those with visible small changes in bone structure to a well-defined radiolucent periapical area, and further increased to 100% for those with severe apical periodontitis [68]. Results from a more recent study were consistent to prior findings, in that sinuses with >2 mm membrane thickening were more likely to have associated teeth with periapical lesions (53.6% versus 42.1%) [69]. The chance of having membrane thickening when there was associated periapical lesions was estimated to be as high as thrice than when there was no periapical lesion [71]. The periapical lesion did not necessarily have to be in contact or enter the sinus floor to elicit sinus membrane thickening [68]. The number of associated root canal treatments also did not influence the degree of thickening [69].

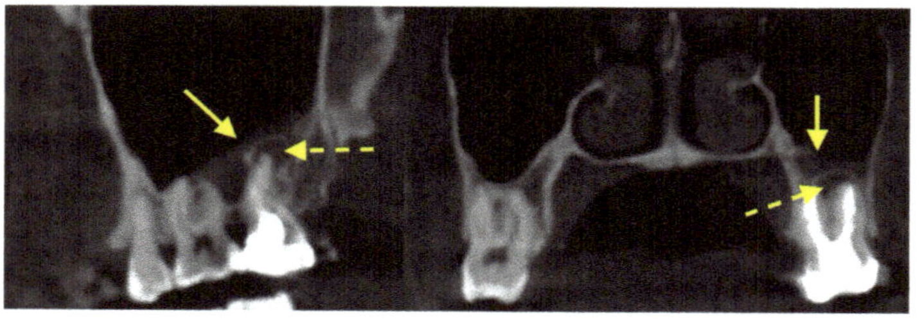

Figure 4. Sinus membrane thickening (solid arrow) in the left maxillary sinus associated with a periapical lesion (dotted arrow).

3.2. Membrane Thickening Associated with Periodontal Lesions

Similar to periapical lesions, it seemed that membrane thickening was more prevalent when the associated teeth has more severe periodontal bone loss. The chance of membrane thickening for those with severe periodontal bone loss was 4.6 times than those with mild bone loss [72]. Those with class II or class III furcation lesions were 1.6 and 3.5 times, respectively, more likely to have membrane thickening than those without furcation involvement [72]. The presence of vertical intrabony pockets also led to membrane thickening being 2.4–5.6 times more likely than without such pockets [72]. The extraction of the periodontally involved tooth would lead to the complete resolution of the membrane thickening at 4 months [73]. For a comprehensive review on the effect of periapical and periodontal pathologies on membrane thickening, readers can refer to [74].

3.3. Mucous Retention Cyst (MRC)

MRCs are commonly found in the maxillary sinus (Figure 5). MRCs were found in 10.1– 28.6% of the maxillary sinus [28,75–77]. Up to four MRCs were reported within a single sinus [75,77]. MRCs were more commonly located at the sinus walls (19.9–53.6%) and the floor (28.6–76.7%) instead of the roof (3.4–17.9%) [75,77]. The average size of an MRC was reported to be 551 ± 1368 mm^3 with a diameter of 9.6 ± 5.4 mm [76]. The presence of MRCs on the sinus floor was more likely if there were teeth with periapical lesions, were endodontically treated, or with severe bone loss [76,77].

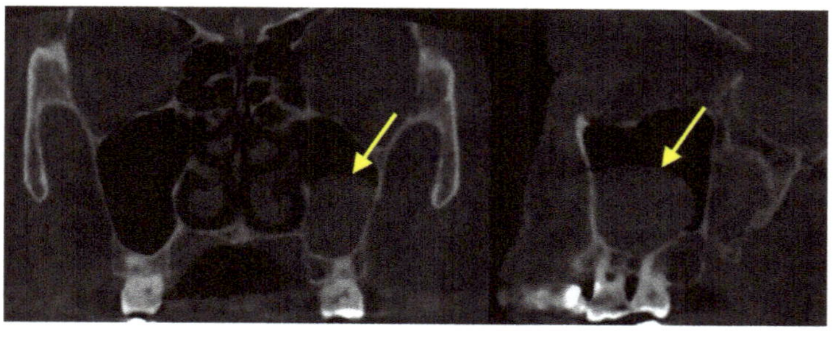

Figure 5. Mucous retention cyst in the left maxillary sinus.

3.4. Antrolith

Antrolith is a calcified mass in the maxillary sinus (Figure 6). Antroliths were found in 0.6–8.4% of maxillary sinuses [42,78,79]. They could be punctate (14.3–53.1%), linear (31.4–34.3%), or amorphous (15.5–22.9%) [78,80]. Most of them were located at the molar region (95.0%) rather than the premolar region (5.0%), and located in the sinus floor (62.9–77.5%) [79,80]. The size of an antrolith was found to be between 1–91 mm^2, as measured by the maximum cross-sectional area computed from the coronal slices [78]. Another study reported the mean length was 5.6 $\pm$ 4.4 mm, width was 4.1 $\pm$ 2.9 mm, and height was 3.5 $\pm$ 2.1 mm [79]. Intuitively, the presence of antroliths might seem to pose an increased risk of membrane perforation following implant insertion with simultaneous sinus floor elevation, but study results did not find such increased risk [81].

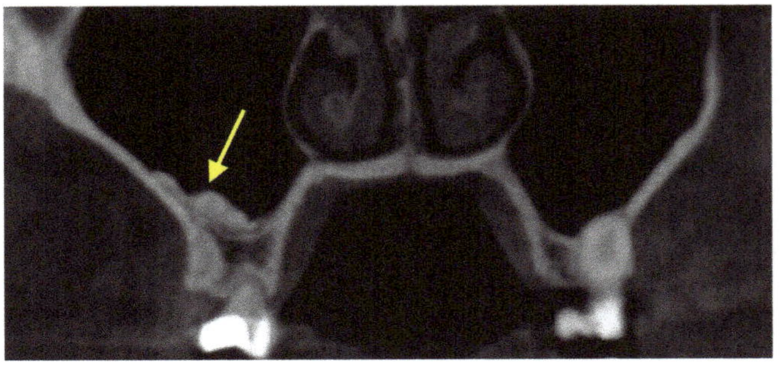

Figure 6. Antrolith found on the sinus floor of the right maxillary sinus.

3.5. Foreign Bodies

Due to the proximity of the maxillary sinus floor with the dentoalveolar region, iatrogenic introduction of foreign bodies into the sinus can sometimes occur. The foreign bodies can be localized with the aid of CBCT imaging. For example, one study reported 27 patients with foreign bodies introduced into their maxillary sinus, including tooth fragments, complete teeth, dental implants, dental impression material, root filling material, and dental bur [82]. Ample root filling material could be pushed into the maxillary sinus through a perforated root during root canal treatment [83]. Meanwhile, it was found that most of the cases with dental implants introduced into the sinus did not receive a presurgical CBCT exam even in the presence of a severely atrophic edentulous ridge [84]. One uncommon foreign body was a metallic hand sewing needle inserted by a patient into a cavitated tooth to remove trapped food debris, which subsequently disappeared and found to be pushed into the maxillary sinus as confirmed by CBCT [85]. Orthodontic mini-screws might also intrude into the sinus particularly if the sinus floor is <6.0 mm to the alveolar ridge crest [86].

4. Artificial Intelligence in Sinus Diagnosis

Nowadays, there are many research works on artificial intelligence including machine learning that can help clinicians detect abnormal findings in the maxillary sinus from CBCT images [87]. To begin with, convolutional neural network (CNN) could be used to automatically segment the maxillary sinus into the bone, air and lesion [88,89], such as MRC [90] or even complete opacification [91]. CNN could also be used to classify if a maxillary sinus was healthy or with sinusitis [92], and to detect the location of the maxillary sinus floor and automatically measure the associated alveolar ridge height for implant planning [93]. In addition, maxillary sinus features, such as sinus volume or linear measurements, were proven to be useful in dental age assessment and sex identification based on CBCT images [94,95]. Meanwhile, CBCT image filter driven by artificial intelligence has been developed to enhance the visualization of the maxillary sinus anatomy for various diagnostic purposes, such as to evaluate sinus membrane thickening associated with periapical lesions [96].

5. Conclusions

The use of CBCT is becoming more and more common in dental practice. The maxillary sinuses can be visualized by CBCT in a medium-to-large field-of-view volume that covers the maxillofacial region. The visualization and assessment of the maxillary sinus is very important prior to procedures that take place in close proximity with the sinus floor, such as tooth extraction, implant insertion, and sinus floor elevation. Some sinus pathologies may be associated with odontogenic lesions, such as periapical diseases and periodontal bone loss. The maxillary sinus may also involve other pathologies, such as fungal infections, allergic pathologies, benign and malignant lesions, and trauma. Clinicians should be familiar with the common anatomical features and sinus pathologies, to facilitate better diagnosis and treatment planning, and promptly refer patients to the oral and maxillofacial surgeons to follow up if needed. This review briefly covered the common and clinically relevant anatomical and pathological features concerning the maxillary sinus. It was intended to increase the awareness of the clinicians about the relevance of sinus health and pathology to clinical dentistry. To recap, the following anatomical features were reviewed: PSAA and lateral wall thickness, sinus pneumatization, sinus hypoplasia, sinus augmentation, sinus septa, and primary and accessory ostia. The following pathological features were reviewed: sinus membrane thickening associated with periapical and periodontal lesions, MRC, antrolith, and foreign bodies. The latest development in artificial intelligence in sinus diagnosis was also covered. Certainly, the features covered were not exhaustive, and readers should refer to specialized oral and maxillofacial radiology textbooks for a comprehensive description of all relevant features and proper image interpretation regarding the maxillary sinus.

Author Contributions: A.W.K.Y.; writing—original draft preparation, K.F.H., D.T.S.L. and Y.Y.L.; writing—review and editing. All authors have read and agreed to the published version of the manuscript.

Funding: This research received no external funding.

Institutional Review Board Statement: Not applicable.

Informed Consent Statement: Not applicable.

Data Availability Statement: Not applicable.

Conflicts of Interest: The authors declare no conflict of interest.

References

1. Martu, C.; Martu, M.-A.; Maftei, G.-A.; Diaconu-Popa, D.A.; Radulescu, L. Odontogenic Sinusitis: From Diagnosis to Treatment Possibilities—A Narrative Review of Recent Data. *Diagnostics* **2022**, *12*, 1600. [CrossRef] [PubMed]
2. Braun, M.J.; Rauneker, T.; Dreyhaupt, J.; Hoffmann, T.K.; Luthardt, R.G.; Schmitz, B.; Dammann, F.; Beer, M. Dental and Maxillofacial Cone Beam CT—High Number of Incidental Findings and Their Impact on Follow-Up and Therapy Management. *Diagnostics* **2022**, *12*, 1036. [CrossRef] [PubMed]
3. Lopes, L.J.; Gamba, T.O.; Bertinato, J.V.; Freitas, D.Q. Comparison of panoramic radiography and CBCT to identify maxillary posterior roots invading the maxillary sinus. *Dentomaxillofac. Radiol.* **2016**, *45*, 20160043. [CrossRef] [PubMed]
4. Sun, W.; Xia, K.; Tang, L.; Liu, C.; Zou, L.; Liu, J. Accuracy of panoramic radiography in diagnosing maxillary sinus-root relationship: A systematic review and meta-analysis. *Angle Orthod.* **2018**, *88*, 819–829. [CrossRef]
5. Kirkham-Ali, K.; La, M.; Sher, J.; Sholapurkar, A. Comparison of cone-beam computed tomography and panoramic imaging in assessing the relationship between posterior maxillary tooth roots and the maxillary sinus: A systematic review. *J. Investig. Clin. Dent.* **2019**, *10*, e12402. [CrossRef]
6. Constantine, S.; Clark, B.; Kiermeier, A.; Anderson, P. Panoramic radiography is of limited value in the evaluation of maxillary sinus disease. *Oral Surg. Oral Med. Oral Pathol. Oral Radiol.* **2019**, *127*, 237–246. [CrossRef]
7. Lang, A.; Schulze, R. Detection accuracy of maxillary sinus floor septa in panoramic radiographs using CBCT as gold standard: A multi-observer receiver operating characteristic (ROC) study. *Clin. Oral Investig.* **2019**, *23*, 99–105. [CrossRef]

8. Vollmer, A.; Saravi, B.; Vollmer, M.; Lang, G.M.; Straub, A.; Brands, R.C.; Kübler, A.; Gubik, S.; Hartmann, S. Artificial Intelligence-Based Prediction of Oroantral Communication after Tooth Extraction Utilizing Preoperative Panoramic Radiography. *Diagnostics* **2022**, *12*, 1406. [CrossRef]
9. Sekerci, A.E.; Sisman, Y.; Etoz, M.; Bulut, D.G. Aberrant anatomical variation of maxillary sinus mimicking periapical cyst: A report of two cases and role of CBCT in diagnosis. *Case Rep. Dent.* **2013**, *2013*, 757645. [CrossRef]
10. Yeung, A.W.K. Seminal Works and Historical Roots of Dental Implant Research with the Use of CBCT. *Int. J. Oral Maxillofac. Implant.* **2021**, *36*, 731–736. [CrossRef]
11. Huang, X.; Bai, J.; Liu, X.; Meng, Z.; Shang, Y.; Jiao, T.; Chen, G.; Deng, J. Scientometric analysis of dental implant research over the past 10 years and future research trends. *BioMed Res. Int.* **2021**, *2021*, 6634055. [CrossRef] [PubMed]
12. Brown, J.; Jacobs, R.; Levring Jäghagen, E.; Lindh, C.; Baksi, G.; Schulze, D.; Schulze, R. Basic training requirements for the use of dental CBCT by dentists: A position paper prepared by the European Academy of DentoMaxilloFacial Radiology. *Dentomaxillofac. Radiol.* **2014**, *43*, 20130291. [CrossRef] [PubMed]
13. Vogiatzi, T.; Kloukos, D.; Scarfe, W.C.; Bornstein, M.M. Incidence of anatomical variations and disease of the maxillary sinuses as identified by cone beam computed tomography: A systematic review. *Int. J. Oral Maxillofac. Implant.* **2014**, *29*, 1301–1314. [CrossRef] [PubMed]
14. Hung, K.F.; Hui, L.L.; Leung, Y.Y. Patient-specific estimation of the bone graft volume needed for maxillary sinus floor elevation: A radiographic study using cone-beam computed tomography. *Clin. Oral Investig.* **2022**, *26*, 3875–3884. [CrossRef]
15. Benavides, E.; Rios, H.F.; Ganz, S.D.; An, C.-H.; Resnik, R.; Reardon, G.T.; Feldman, S.J.; Mah, J.K.; Hatcher, D.; Kim, M.-J. Use of cone beam computed tomography in implant dentistry: The International Congress of Oral Implantologists consensus report. *Implant Dent.* **2012**, *21*, 78–86. [CrossRef]
16. Bornstein, M.M.; Scarfe, W.C.; Vaughn, V.M.; Jacobs, R. Cone beam computed tomography in implant dentistry: A systematic review focusing on guidelines, indications, and radiation dose risks. *Int. J. Oral Maxillofac. Implant.* **2014**, *29*, 55–77. [CrossRef]
17. Harris, D.; Horner, K.; Gröndahl, K.; Jacobs, R.; Helmrot, E.; Benic, G.I.; Bornstein, M.M.; Dawood, A.; Quirynen, M. EAO guidelines for the use of diagnostic imaging in implant dentistry 2011. A consensus workshop organized by the European Association for Osseointegration at the Medical University of Warsaw. *Clin. Oral Implant. Res.* **2012**, *23*, 1243–1253. [CrossRef]
18. Kusnoto, B.; Kaur, P.; Salem, A.; Zhang, Z.; Galang-Boquiren, M.T.; Viana, G.; Evans, C.A.; Manasse, R.; Monahan, R.; BeGole, E. Implementation of ultra-low-dose CBCT for routine 2D orthodontic diagnostic radiographs: Cephalometric landmark identification and image quality assessment. *Semin. Orthod.* **2015**, *21*, 233–247. [CrossRef]
19. Rigolone, M.; Pasqualini, D.; Bianchi, L.; Berutti, E.; Bianchi, S.D. Vestibular surgical access to the palatine root of the superior first molar:"low-dose cone-beam" CT analysis of the pathway and its anatomic variations. *J. Endod.* **2003**, *29*, 773–775. [CrossRef]
20. Chindasombatjaroen, J.; Poomsawat, S.; Klongnoi, B. Calcifying cystic odontogenic tumor associated with other lesions: Case report with cone-beam computed tomography findings. *Oral Surg. Oral Med. Oral Pathol. Oral Radiol.* **2012**, *113*, 414–420. [CrossRef]
21. Yeung, A.W.K. The "As Low As Reasonably Achievable" (ALARA) principle: A brief historical overview and a bibliometric analysis of the most cited publications. *Radioprotection* **2019**, *54*, 103–109. [CrossRef]
22. Jaju, P.P.; Jaju, S.P. Cone-beam computed tomography: Time to move from ALARA to ALADA. *Imaging Sci. Dent.* **2015**, *45*, 263–265. [CrossRef] [PubMed]
23. Oenning, A.C.; Jacobs, R.; Salmon, B. ALADAIP, beyond ALARA and towards personalized optimization for paediatric cone-beam CT. *Int. J. Paediatr. Dent.* **2021**, *31*, 676–678. [CrossRef] [PubMed]
24. Hung, K.F.; Hui, L.; Yeung, A.W.K.; Jacobs, R.; Leung, Y.Y.; Bornstein, M.M. An analysis of patient dose received during cone-beam computed tomography in relation to scan settings and imaging indications as seen in a dental institution in order to establish institutional diagnostic reference levels. *Dentomaxillofac. Radiol.* **2022**, *51*, 20200529. [CrossRef] [PubMed]
25. Yeung, A.W.K.; Wong, N.S.M. Reject Rates of Radiographic Images in Dentomaxillofacial Radiology: A Literature Review. *Int. J. Environ. Res. Public Health* **2021**, *18*, 8076. [CrossRef]
26. Hung, K.; Hui, L.; Yeung, A.W.K.; Scarfe, W.C.; Bornstein, M.M. Image retake rates of cone beam computed tomography in a dental institution. *Clin. Oral Investig.* **2020**, *24*, 4501–4510. [CrossRef]
27. Beale, T.J.; Madani, G.; Morley, S.J. Imaging of the paranasal sinuses and nasal cavity: Normal anatomy and clinically relevant anatomical variants. *Semin. Ultrasound CT MRI* **2009**, *30*, 2–16. [CrossRef]
28. Rege, I.C.C.; Sousa, T.O.; Leles, C.R.; Mendonça, E.F. Occurrence of maxillary sinus abnormalities detected by cone beam CT in asymptomatic patients. *BMC Oral Health* **2012**, *12*, 30. [CrossRef]
29. Ella, B.; Sédarat, C.; Da Costa Noble, R.; Normand, E.; Lauverjat, Y.; Siberchicot, F.; Caix, P.; Zwetyenga, N. Vascular connections of the lateral wall of the sinus: Surgical effect in sinus augmentation. *Int. J. Oral Maxillofac. Implant.* **2008**, *23*, 1047–1052.
30. Jensen, S.S.; Eriksen, J.; Schiodt, M. Severe bleeding after sinus floor elevation using the transcrestal technique: A case report. *Eur. J. Oral Implant.* **2012**, *5*, 287–291.
31. Ilgüy, D.; Ilgüy, M.; Dolekoglu, S.; Fisekcioglu, E. Evaluation of the posterior superior alveolar artery and the maxillary sinus with CBCT. *Braz. Oral Res.* **2013**, *27*, 431–437. [CrossRef] [PubMed]
32. Tehranchi, M.; Taleghani, F.; Shahab, S.; Nouri, A. Prevalence and location of the posterior superior alveolar artery using cone-beam computed tomography. *Imaging Sci. Dent.* **2017**, *47*, 39–44. [CrossRef] [PubMed]

33. Danesh-Sani, S.A.; Movahed, A.; ElChaar, E.S.; Chong Chan, K.; Amintavakoli, N. Radiographic evaluation of maxillary sinus lateral wall and posterior superior alveolar artery anatomy: A cone-beam computed tomographic study. *Clin. Implant Dent. Relat. Res.* **2017**, *19*, 151–160. [CrossRef]
34. Jung, J.; Yim, J.-H.; Kwon, Y.-D.; Al-Nawas, B.; Kim, G.-T.; Choi, B.-J.; Lee, D.-W. A radiographic study of the position and prevalence of the maxillary arterial endosseous anastomosis using cone beam computed tomography. *Int. J. Oral Maxillofac. Implant.* **2011**, *26*, 1273–1278.
35. Lozano-Carrascal, N.; Salomó-Coll, O.; Gehrke, S.A.; Calvo-Guirado, J.L.; Hernández-Alfaro, F.; Gargallo-Albiol, J. Radiological evaluation of maxillary sinus anatomy: A cross-sectional study of 300 patients. *Ann. Anat. -Anat. Anz.* **2017**, *214*, 1–8. [CrossRef]
36. Ang, K.-Y.; Ang, K.-L.; Ngeow, W.C. The prevalence and location of the posterior superior alveolar artery in the maxillary sinus wall: A preliminary computed-cone beam study. *Saudi Dent. J.* **2022**, *34*, 629–635. [CrossRef] [PubMed]
37. Varela-Centelles, P.; Loira-Gago, M.; Seoane-Romero, J.; Takkouche, B.; Monteiro, L.; Seoane, J. Detection of the posterior superior alveolar artery in the lateral sinus wall using computed tomography/cone beam computed tomography: A prevalence meta-analysis study and systematic review. *Int. J. Oral Maxillofac. Surg.* **2015**, *44*, 1405–1410. [CrossRef]
38. Basma, H.; Saleh, I.; Abou-Arraj, R.; Li, P.; Benavides, E.; Wang, H.-L.; Chang, H.-L. Association between lateral wall thickness and sinus membrane perforation during lateral sinus elevation: A retrospective study. *Int. J. Oral Implant* **2021**, *14*, 77–85.
39. Kiakojori, A.; Nasab, S.P.M.; Abesi, F.; Gholinia, H. Radiographic assessment of maxillary sinus lateral wall thickness in edentulous posterior maxilla. *Electron. Physician* **2017**, *9*, 5948–5953. [CrossRef]
40. Lim, E.L.; Ngeow, W.C.; Lim, D. The implications of different lateral wall thicknesses on surgical access to the maxillary sinus. *Braz. Oral Res.* **2017**, *31*, e97. [CrossRef]
41. Rahpeyma, A.; Khajehahmadi, S.; Amini, P. Alveolar antral artery: Does its diameter correlate with maxillary lateral wall thickness in dentate patients? *Iran. J. Otorhinolaryngol.* **2014**, *26*, 163–167. [PubMed]
42. Pelinsari Lana, J.; Moura Rodrigues Carneiro, P.; de Carvalho Machado, V.; Eduardo Alencar de Souza, P.; Ricardo Manzi, F.; Campolina Rebello Horta, M. Anatomic variations and lesions of the maxillary sinus detected in cone beam computed tomography for dental implants. *Clin. Oral Implant. Res.* **2012**, *23*, 1398–1403. [CrossRef]
43. Cavalcanti, M.C.; Guirado, T.E.; Sapata, V.M.; Costa, C.; Pannuti, C.M.; Jung, R.E.; César Neto, J.B. Maxillary sinus floor pneumatization and alveolar ridge resorption after tooth loss: A cross-sectional study. *Braz. Oral Res.* **2018**, *32*, e64. [CrossRef] [PubMed]
44. Wu, X.; Cai, Q.; Huang, D.; Xiong, P.; Shi, L. Cone-beam computed tomography-based analysis of maxillary sinus pneumatization extended into the alveolar process in different age groups. *BMC Oral Health* **2022**, *22*, 393. [CrossRef]
45. Hamdy, R.M. Three-dimensional linear and volumetric analysis of maxillary sinus pneumatization. *J. Adv. Res.* **2014**, *5*, 387–395. [CrossRef]
46. Lombardi, T.; Bernardello, F.; Berton, F.; Porrelli, D.; Rapani, A.; Camurri Piloni, A.; Fiorillo, L.; Di Lenarda, R.; Stacchi, C. Efficacy of alveolar ridge preservation after maxillary molar extraction in reducing crestal bone resorption and sinus pneumatization: A multicenter prospective case-control study. *BioMed Res. Int.* **2018**, *2018*, 9352130. [CrossRef] [PubMed]
47. Günaçar, D.N.; Köse, T.E.; Arsan, B.; Aydın, E.Z. Radioanatomic study of maxillary sinus palatal process pneumatization. *Oral Radiol.* **2022**, *38*, 398–404. [CrossRef]
48. Alsufyani, N.; El-Hakim, H.; Major, P. Prevalence of maxillary sinus hypoplasia and association with variations in the sinonasal complex: A cone beam CT study. *Clin. Oral Investig.* **2021**, *25*, 5463–5471. [CrossRef]
49. Allareddy, V.; Vincent, S.D.; Hellstein, J.W.; Qian, F.; Smoker, W.R.; Ruprecht, A. Incidental findings on cone beam computed tomography images. *Int. J. Dent.* **2012**, *2012*, 871532. [CrossRef]
50. Jafari-Pozve, N.; Sheikhi, M.; Ataie-Khorasgani, M.; Jafari-Pozve, S. Aplasia and hypoplasia of the maxillary sinus: A case series. *Dent. Res. J.* **2014**, *11*, 615–617.
51. Alsufyani, N.A.; Major, M.P.; Major, P.W. Relationship between maxillary sinus hypoplasia and maxillary occlusal cant: A cone beam CT study. *BioMed Res. Int.* **2021**, *2022*, 4651514. [CrossRef]
52. Klijn, R.; Van Den Beucken, J.; Bronkhorst, E.; Berge, S.; Meijer, G.; Jansen, J. Predictive value of ridge dimensions on autologous bone graft resorption in staged maxillary sinus augmentation surgery using Cone-Beam CT. *Clin. Oral Implant. Res.* **2012**, *23*, 409–415. [CrossRef] [PubMed]
53. Okada, T.; Kanai, T.; Tachikawa, N.; Munakata, M.; Kasugai, S. Long-term radiographic assessment of maxillary sinus floor augmentation using beta-tricalcium phosphate: Analysis by cone-beam computed tomography. *Int. J. Implant Dent.* **2016**, *2*, 8. [CrossRef] [PubMed]
54. Kivovics, M.; Szabó, B.T.; Németh, O.; Iványi, D.; Trimmel, B.; Szmirnova, I.; Orhan, K.; Mijiritsky, E.; Szabó, G.; Dobó-Nagy, C. Comparison between micro-computed tomography and cone-beam computed tomography in the assessment of bone quality and a long-term volumetric study of the augmented sinus grafted with an albumin impregnated allograft. *J. Clin. Med.* **2020**, *9*, 303. [CrossRef] [PubMed]
55. Kwon, J.J.; Hwang, J.; Kim, Y.D.; Shin, S.H.; Cho, B.H.; Lee, J.Y. Automatic three-dimensional analysis of bone volume and quality change after maxillary sinus augmentation. *Clin. Implant Dent. Relat. Res.* **2019**, *21*, 1148–1155. [CrossRef] [PubMed]
56. Soardi, C.M.; Zaffe, D.; Motroni, A.; Wang, H.L. Quantitative comparison of cone beam computed tomography and microradiography in the evaluation of bone density after maxillary sinus augmentation: A preliminary study. *Clin. Implant Dent. Relat. Res.* **2014**, *16*, 557–564. [CrossRef]

57. Bornstein, M.M.; Seiffert, C.; Maestre-Ferrín, L.; Fodich, I.; Jacobs, R.; Buser, D.; von Arx, T. An Analysis of Frequency, Morphology, and Locations of Maxillary Sinus Septa Using Cone Beam Computed Tomography. *Int. J. Oral Maxillofac. Implant.* **2016**, *31*, 280–287. [CrossRef]
58. Tadinada, A.; Jalali, E.; Al-Salman, W.; Jambhekar, S.; Katechia, B.; Almas, K. Prevalence of bony septa, antral pathology, and dimensions of the maxillary sinus from a sinus augmentation perspective: A retrospective cone-beam computed tomography study. *Imaging Sci. Dent.* **2016**, *46*, 109–115. [CrossRef]
59. Hungerbühler, A.; Rostetter, C.; Lübbers, H.-T.; Rücker, M.; Stadlinger, B. Anatomical characteristics of maxillary sinus septa visualized by cone beam computed tomography. *Int. J. Oral Maxillofac. Surg.* **2019**, *48*, 382–387. [CrossRef]
60. Orhan, K.; Seker, B.K.; Aksoy, S.; Bayindir, H.; Berberoğlu, A.; Seker, E. Cone beam CT evaluation of maxillary sinus septa prevalence, height, location and morphology in children and an adult population. *Med. Princ. Pract.* **2013**, *22*, 47–53. [CrossRef]
61. Sigaroudi, A.K.; Kajan, Z.D.; Rastgar, S.; Asli, H.N. Frequency of different maxillary sinus septal patterns found on cone-beam computed tomography and predicting the associated risk of sinus membrane perforation during sinus lifting. *Imaging Sci. Dent.* **2017**, *47*, 261–267. [CrossRef] [PubMed]
62. Shanbhag, S.; Karnik, P.; Shirke, P.; Shanbhag, V. Cone-beam computed tomographic analysis of sinus membrane thickness, ostium patency, and residual ridge heights in the posterior maxilla: Implications for sinus floor elevation. *Clin. Oral Implant. Res.* **2014**, *25*, 755–760. [CrossRef] [PubMed]
63. Guo, Z.Z.; Liu, Y.; Qin, L.; Song, Y.L.; Xie, C.; Li, D.H. Longitudinal response of membrane thickness and ostium patency following sinus floor elevation: A prospective cohort study. *Clin. Oral Implant. Res.* **2016**, *27*, 724–729. [CrossRef] [PubMed]
64. Yeung, A.W.K.; Colsoul, N.; Montalvao, C.; Hung, K.; Jacobs, R.; Bornstein, M.M. Visibility, location, and morphology of the primary maxillary sinus ostium and presence of accessory ostia: A retrospective analysis using cone beam computed tomography (CBCT). *Clin. Oral Investig.* **2019**, *23*, 3977–3986. [CrossRef] [PubMed]
65. Hung, K.; Montalvao, C.; Yeung, A.W.K.; Li, G.; Bornstein, M.M. Frequency, location, and morphology of accessory maxillary sinus ostia: A retrospective study using cone beam computed tomography (CBCT). *Surg. Radiol. Anat.* **2020**, *42*, 219–228. [CrossRef]
66. Ali, I.K.; Sansare, K.; Karjodkar, F.R.; Vanga, K.; Salve, P.; Pawar, A.M. Cone-beam computed tomography analysis of accessory maxillary ostium and Haller cells: Prevalence and clinical significance. *Imaging Sci. Dent.* **2017**, *47*, 33–37. [CrossRef]
67. Shetty, S.; Al Bayatti, S.W.; Al-Rawi, N.H.; Samsudin, R.; Marei, H.; Shetty, R.; Abdelmagyd, H.A.; Reddy, S. A study on the association between accessory maxillary ostium and maxillary sinus mucosal thickening using cone beam computed tomography. *Head Face Med.* **2021**, *17*, 28. [CrossRef]
68. Lu, Y.; Liu, Z.; Zhang, L.; Zhou, X.; Zheng, Q.; Duan, X.; Zheng, G.; Wang, H.; Huang, D. Associations between maxillary sinus mucosal thickening and apical periodontitis using cone-beam computed tomography scanning: A retrospective study. *J. Endod.* **2012**, *38*, 1069–1074. [CrossRef]
69. Aksoy, U.; Orhan, K. Association between odontogenic conditions and maxillary sinus mucosal thickening: A retrospective CBCT study. *Clin. Oral Investig.* **2019**, *23*, 123–131. [CrossRef] [PubMed]
70. Bornstein, M.M.; Wasmer, J.; Sendi, P.; Janner, S.F.; Buser, D.; Von Arx, T. Characteristics and dimensions of the Schneiderian membrane and apical bone in maxillary molars referred for apical surgery: A comparative radiographic analysis using limited cone beam computed tomography. *J. Endod.* **2012**, *38*, 51–57. [CrossRef] [PubMed]
71. Nascimento, E.H.L.; Pontual, M.L.A.; Pontual, A.A.; Freitas, D.Q.; Perez, D.E.C.; Ramos-Perez, F.M. Association between odontogenic conditions and maxillary sinus disease: A study using cone-beam computed tomography. *J. Endod.* **2016**, *42*, 1509–1515. [CrossRef] [PubMed]
72. Ren, S.; Zhao, H.; Liu, J.; Wang, Q.; Pan, Y. Significance of maxillary sinus mucosal thickening in patients with periodontal disease. *Int. Dent. J.* **2015**, *65*, 303–310. [CrossRef]
73. Cao, Z.; Yuan, J. Changes in Maxillary Sinus Mucosal Thickening following the Extraction of Teeth with Advanced Periodontal Disease: A Retrospective Study Using Cone-Beam Computed Tomography. *BioMed Res. Int.* **2021**, *2021*, 6688634. [CrossRef] [PubMed]
74. Eggmann, F.; Connert, T.; Bühler, J.; Dagassan-Berndt, D.; Weiger, R.; Walter, C. Do periapical and periodontal pathologies affect Schneiderian membrane appearance? Systematic review of studies using cone-beam computed tomography. *Clin. Oral Investig.* **2017**, *21*, 1611–1630. [CrossRef] [PubMed]
75. Yeung, A.W.K.; Tanaka, R.; Khong, P.-L.; von Arx, T.; Bornstein, M.M. Frequency, location, and association with dental pathology of mucous retention cysts in the maxillary sinus. A radiographic study using cone beam computed tomography (CBCT). *Clin. Oral Investig.* **2018**, *22*, 1175–1183. [CrossRef] [PubMed]
76. Hung, K.; Hui, L.; Yeung, A.W.K.; Wu, Y.; Hsung, R.T.-C.; Bornstein, M.M. Volumetric analysis of mucous retention cysts in the maxillary sinus: A retrospective study using cone-beam computed tomography. *Imaging Sci. Dent.* **2021**, *51*, 117–127. [CrossRef]
77. Ren, L.; Chen, C.; Li, N.; Hu, J.; Jiang, Z.; Yang, G. Prevalence of and factors associated with maxillary sinus cyst in a Chinese population. *J. Oral Sci.* **2022**, *64*, 22–27. [CrossRef] [PubMed]
78. Cho, B.-H.; Jung, Y.-H.; Hwang, J.-J. Maxillary antroliths detected by cone-beam computed tomography in an adult dental population. *Imaging Sci. Dent.* **2019**, *49*, 59–63. [CrossRef]

79. Chen, H.-H.; Yi, C.-A.; Chen, Y.-C.; Huang, H.-H. Anatomical characteristics of maxillary sinus antroliths and their influence on sinus membrane thickness: A retrospective cone beam computed tomography analysis. *Int. J. Oral Maxillofac. Surg.* **2021**, *50*, 1107–1112. [CrossRef]
80. Kawai, T.; Tanaka, R.; Yeung, A.W.K.; von Arx, T.; Bornstein, M.M. Frequency and type of incidentally detected radiodensities in the maxillary sinus: A retrospective analysis using cone beam computed tomography (CBCT). *Clin. Oral Investig.* **2019**, *23*, 1091–1099. [CrossRef]
81. Chen, H.H.; Yi, C.A.; Chen, Y.C.; Tsai, C.C.; Lin, P.Y.; Huang, H.H. Influence of maxillary antrolith on the clinical outcome of implants placed simultaneously with osteotome sinus floor elevation: A retrospective radiographic study. *Clin. Implant Dent. Relat. Res.* **2021**, *23*, 833–841. [CrossRef] [PubMed]
82. Tilaveridis, I.; Stefanidou, A.; Kyrgidis, A.; Tilaveridis, S.; Tilaveridou, S.; Zouloumis, L. Foreign Bodies of Dental Iatrogenic Origin Displaced in the Maxillary Sinus-A Safety and Efficacy Analysis of a Retrospective Study. *Ann. Maxillofac. Surg.* **2022**, *12*, 33–38. [PubMed]
83. Rahnama, M.; Łobacz, M.; Kiełbowicz, D.; Grasza, J. Foreign body in the maxillary sinus–a case report. *Curr. Issues Pharm. Med. Sci.* **2012**, *25*, 15–17. [CrossRef]
84. Sgaramella, N.; Tartaro, G.; D'Amato, S.; Santagata, M.; Colella, G. Displacement of dental implants into the maxillary sinus: A retrospective study of twenty-one patients. *Clin. Implant Dent. Relat. Res.* **2016**, *18*, 62–72. [CrossRef] [PubMed]
85. Shao, L.; Qin, X.; Ma, Y. Removal of maxillary sinus metallic foreign body like a hand sewing needle by magnetic iron. *Int. J. Clin. Pediatric Dent.* **2014**, *7*, 61–64. [CrossRef]
86. Motoyoshi, M.; Sanuki-Suzuki, R.; Uchida, Y.; Saiki, A.; Shimizu, N. Maxillary sinus perforation by orthodontic anchor screws. *J. Oral Sci.* **2015**, *57*, 95–100. [CrossRef]
87. Patil, S.; Albogami, S.; Hosmani, J.; Mujoo, S.; Kamil, M.A.; Mansour, M.A.; Abdul, H.N.; Bhandi, S.; Ahmed, S.S. Artificial Intelligence in the Diagnosis of Oral Diseases: Applications and Pitfalls. *Diagnostics* **2022**, *12*, 1029. [CrossRef]
88. Jung, S.-K.; Lim, H.-K.; Lee, S.; Cho, Y.; Song, I.-S. Deep active learning for automatic segmentation of maxillary sinus lesions using a convolutional neural network. *Diagnostics* **2021**, *11*, 688. [CrossRef]
89. Morgan, N.; Van Gerven, A.; Smolders, A.; de Faria Vasconcelos, K.; Willems, H.; Jacobs, R. Convolutional neural network for automatic maxillary sinus segmentation on cone-beam computed tomographic images. *Sci. Rep.* **2022**, *12*, 7523. [CrossRef]
90. Hung, K.F.; Ai, Q.Y.H.; King, A.D.; Bornstein, M.M.; Wong, L.M.; Leung, Y.Y. Automatic detection and segmentation of morphological changes of the maxillary sinus mucosa on cone-beam computed tomography images using a three-dimensional convolutional neural network. *Clin. Oral Investig.* **2022**, *26*, 3987–3998. [CrossRef]
91. Choi, H.; Jeon, K.J.; Kim, Y.H.; Ha, E.-G.; Lee, C.; Han, S.-S. Deep learning-based fully automatic segmentation of the maxillary sinus on cone-beam computed tomographic images. *Sci. Rep.* **2022**, *12*, 14009. [CrossRef] [PubMed]
92. Serindere, G.; Bilgili, E.; Yesil, C.; Ozveren, N. Evaluation of maxillary sinusitis from panoramic radiographs and cone-beam computed tomographic images using a convolutional neural network. *Imaging Sci. Dent.* **2022**, *52*, 187–195. [CrossRef] [PubMed]
93. Kurt Bayrakdar, S.; Orhan, K.; Bayrakdar, I.S.; Bilgir, E.; Ezhov, M.; Gusarev, M.; Shumilov, E. A deep learning approach for dental implant planning in cone-beam computed tomography images. *BMC Med. Imaging* **2021**, *21*, 86. [CrossRef] [PubMed]
94. Al-Amodi, A.; Kamel, I.; Al-Rawi, N.H.; Uthman, A.; Shetty, S. Accuracy of Linear Measurements of Maxillary Sinus Dimensions in Gender Identification Using Machine Learning. In Proceedings of the 2021 14th International Conference on Developments in eSystems Engineering (DeSE), Sharjah, United Arab Emirates, 7–10 December 2021; pp. 407–412.
95. Saric, R.; Kevric, J.; Hadziabdic, N.; Osmanovic, A.; Kadic, M.; Saracevic, M.; Jokic, D.; Rajs, V. Dental age assessment based on CBCT images using machine learning algorithms. *Forensic Sci. Int.* **2022**, *334*, 111245. [CrossRef]
96. Estrela, C.R.; Bueno, M.R.; Estrela, M.R.; Estrela, L.R.; Guedes, O.A.; Azevedo, B.C.; Cintra, L.T.A.; Estrela, C. Frequency and risk factors of maxillary sinusitis of endodontic origin evaluated by a dynamic navigation and a new filter of cone-beam computed tomography. *J. Endod.* **2022**, *48*, 1263–1272. [CrossRef]

diagnostics

MDPI

Article

Comparison between Conventional Modality Versus Cone-Beam Computer Tomography on the Assessment of Vertical Furcation in Molars

Jack Lam [1], Andy Wai Kan Yeung [2], Aneesha Acharya [1,3], Chris Fok [1], Melissa Fok [1] and Georgios Pelekos [1,*]

1 Division of Periodontology and Implant Dentistry, Faculty of Dentistry, The University of Hong Kong, Hong Kong SAR, China
2 Division of Applied Oral Sciences & Community Dental Care, The University of Hong Kong, Hong Kong SAR, China
3 Dr. D.Y. Patil Dental College and Hospital, Pune 411018, Maharashtra, India
* Correspondence: george74@hku.hk

Abstract: This study aimed to assess the accuracy of diagnosis of vertical furcation subclass in molars using periapical radiographs (PAs) and clinical chartings compared against cone-beam computer tomography (CBCT) as the gold standard. The protocol involved examiners with different levels of experience. This retrospective radiographic study retrieved 40 molar teeth with full periodontal chartings, PAs, and CBCT records. Fifteen examiners with different levels of experience evaluated the PAs and periodontal chartings to assess the vertical depth of furcation and, thus, the vertical subclassification. CBCT was used as the gold standard for comparison. The accuracy of vertical furcal depth measured was assessed together with the accuracy of vertical subclassification assignment. The reliability of the conventional diagnostic modality among the examiners was also evaluated. A linear mixed model adjusted for the CBCT vertical furcal depth measurement was constructed to determine if tooth position, horizontal furcation distribution, and examiner experience level affect the bias in the vertical depth of furcation measurement. The reliability of the conventional periodontal diagnostic method in measuring vertical furcal depth was found to be fair, while vertical subclass assignment was moderate. Significantly better reliability during subclass assignment was found with mandibular molars ($p < 0.001$) and in maxillary molars with isolated buccal class II furcation. Within the study's limitations, conventional periodontal diagnostics based on periapical radiographs and clinical periodontal chartings appear to be in poor to fair agreement with CBCT (gold standard) when measuring the vertical depth of furcation. Examiners with the least experience were more prone to bias when estimating the vertical furcal depth.

Keywords: furcation; vertical subclassification; cone-beam computer tomography; periodontal diagnostics

1. Introduction

Advanced periodontal disease may be presented with destruction extending into the furcation area of multirooted teeth, leading to furcation involvement (FI). The classic Hamp classification differentiates FI into different degrees depending on the amount of horizontal loss of periodontal tissue support measured with a graduated Nabers furcation probe [1]. According to previous retrospective studies and systematic reviews, most molars with FI respond well to periodontal therapy and could be maintained successfully if supportive periodontal care is provided [2,3]. In the vertical dimension, FI was classified initially into subclasses A, B, and C, with a vertical loss of attachment of 0–3 mm, 4–6 mm, and more than or equal to 7 mm, respectively [4]. A modification was proposed recently with subclasses A, B, and C redefined as attachment loss extending to the coronal, middle, and apical third of the roots, respectively [5].

The degree of vertical furcation subclassification has been shown to affect molars' long-term prognosis in a retrospective cohort study involving 200 periodontal patients who underwent supportive periodontal care for at least ten years. Ten-year survival rates of 91%, 67%, and 23% were reported for molars with vertical subclasses A, B, and C [5]. In another retrospective study, molars with FI were around five times more likely to be extracted than molars with no FI in the multivariable analysis. This risk was higher when the vertical furcation component was considered [6]. Vertical classification allows for the assessment of the indications for planning different furcation treatment options, such as open flap debridement and resective or regenerative periodontal surgeries. In cases with advanced furcal destruction, periodontal regeneration could increase periodontal support and improve tooth prognosis by reducing the furcation subclassification [7]. Vertical subclassification is vital in determining molars' prognosis, deciding on appropriate treatment, and customising supportive care to aid their long-term retention.

A retrospective study compared baseline probing, bone sounding, and intra-surgical vertical and horizontal measurements of furcation defects in molars that received open flap surgeries [8]. Pre-anesthesia probing was the same in 42% and 47.1% of sites concerning the intra-surgical assessment in the vertical and horizontal dimensions. Bone sounding improved the agreement to 59.5% and 64.2%.

Plain radiographs were shown to be in moderate agreement with intra-surgical measurement in terms of horizontal furcation classification [9]. The use of "furcation arrows" on periapical radiographs as an indicator of the presence of FI was found to be of low sensitivity (38.4%) [10]. However, the reliability and validity of PA radiographs in the vertical assessment of furcation have yet to be determined.

A previous in vitro study has demonstrated high consistency between computer tomography and histological sections in classifying horizontal and vertical FI, with jaw specimens' defects artificially created [11]. Another prospective clinical study involving 20 maxillary molars has demonstrated strong agreement between CBCT and intra-surgical measurements of horizontal furcation degree and vertical bone loss, with a difference of 0.36 mm [12]. Therefore, a high correspondence between CBCT and intra-surgical measurement, which is classically deemed as the gold standard, could be expected [13]. Furthermore, CBCT images have been shown to improve the treatment decision-making process and optimise treatment planning in maxillary molars [14,15]. A recent systematic review that explored the evaluation of FI by different diagnostic methods reported that CBCT displayed the closest agreement with intra-surgical measurements, while the accuracy of all the methods was influenced by the examiner's experience [16].

Despite its high consistency and reliability, CBCT is not routinely performed to assess furcation due to concern with the extra radiation dose imposed, compared to traditional plain radiographs. On the other hand, the acquisition of CBCT images using a low-dose protocol, a shorter exposure time, and a smaller field of view could be performed to minimise the effective radiation dose of CBCT [17]. Therefore, this study aimed to assess if diagnosing vertical furcation subclass in molars using conventional periodontal examination methods is reliable and valid. Additionally, the effects of tooth position, furcation involvement distribution, and examiner experience level were investigated.

2. Materials and Methods

2.1. Study Design and Database Search

The current study is a preliminary, retrospective radiographic study comparing the conventional periodontal diagnostic method and cone-beam computer tomography to assess molar furcation involvement in the vertical dimension. A database search of periodontal patients who received care in the periodontology division was performed by the same single calibrated investigator that performed the clinical measurements (GP) to obtain records of molar teeth that met the inclusion criteria. Forty teeth were selected using a convenience sampling method. The study was approved by the Institutional Review Board of the University of Hong Kong/Hospital Authority Hong Kong West Cluster.

2.2. Inclusion and Exclusion Criteria

The inclusion criteria were (i) maxillary or mandibular molars with at least class II furcation involvement and (ii) 6-point clinical periodontal chartings, periapical radiographs, and CBCT DICOM files. Exclusion criteria in this study include (i) poor X-ray and CBCT quality; (ii) periodontal bone loss beyond the apex; (iii) endodontic/periapical pathology; (iv) cracked tooth syndrome/root fracture; (v) molars with fused roots; (vi) presence of fremitus or secondary occlusal trauma; (vii) presence of distolingual root in mandibular molars; (viii) presence of extra mesiobuccal root in maxillary molars; and (ix) presence of extensive metallic restorations close to the furcation area.

2.3. Radiographic Records

All digital periapical radiographs were taken with Durr digital phosphor plates and exposed with an intraoral X-ray machine, Veraview IX (J. Morita, Tokyo, Japan; exposure settings: 60 kV, 7 mA; exposure times: 0.1–0,2 s). Images were imported into the Durr VistaScan Mini view machine (Durr Dental, Stuttgart, Germany). CBCT scanning was performed with either a Veraview X800 unit (J. Morita, Tokyo, Japan; field of view (FOV, diameter x height): 100 × 80 mm; exposure settings: 100 kV, 5 mA; voxel size: 0.125 mm) or ProMax 3D Classic (Planmeca, Helsinki, Finland; FOV: 100 × 100 mm; exposure settings: 90 kV, 8 mA; voxel size: 0.200 mm). All the radiographic records were evaluated by an experienced dental radiologist (AWKY) from the Department of Oral and Maxillofacial Radiology, Faculty of Dentistry, HKU. Radiographs and CBCT images were evaluated for film bending, tilting/angulation error, contrast and brightness, movement during capture, metallic scattering, and artefacts.

2.4. Gold Standard Assessment

CBCT DICOM files of the molars included were imported into the Romexis Viewer (Version 6.1, Planmeca, Helsinki, Finland) and analysed by two calibrated investigators (P.M.L. and A.W.K.Y.). The horizontal furcation involvement, as shown in the clinical charting, was first confirmed on the CBCT images. An assessment of the vertical bone loss in the furcation was then performed. The CBCT viewer axis was first aligned along the long axis of the tooth at the sagittal section and coronal section. At the axial section, the sagittal and coronal planes were adjusted to intersect the canal orifices of the two roots bounding the concerned furcation involvement (Figure 1). The sites with a deeper vertical furcal depth were chosen. The measurement was made to the nearest 0.1 mm using the linear measurement tool on the Romexis Viewer. The tooth was classified according to the modified vertical furcation subclassification and served as the gold standard. By toggling the CBCT along the adjusted axis, the maximal vertical distance from the furcation fornix to the base of the defect and the length of the shorter root bounding the furcation were measured. The exact measurement was repeated on the other furcation entrance(s) if the subject tooth had more than one class II horizontal FI in the maxillary molars (Figure 2).

2.5. Examiners and Image Analysis

In the last decade, CBCT was introduced in the undergraduate curriculum of this institution (HKU) as a new diagnostic modality with increasing popularity due to its three-dimensional nature. During postgraduate training, further practical and theoretical training takes place so that CBCT usage as a diagnostic and treatment planning tool is enhanced. Fifteen examiners consisting of five specialist periodontists (level 3 experience), five postgraduate trainees in the Department of Periodontology and Implant Dentistry (level 2 experience), and five junior hospital dental officers (level 1 experience) were recruited.

The examiners were briefed on the study procedures and the furcation classification systems used in the assessment. Each examiner was provided with clinical periodontal chartings and periapical radiographs. All periapical radiographs were imported into the Romexis Viewer software (Planmeca) and were analysed on the same computer screen (Microsoft Surface Pro 7). On the periapical radiographs, the examiners were asked to measure the vertical bone loss in the furcation area (to the nearest 0.1 mm) using the linear measurement tool in Romexis Viewer with the clinical periodontal charting as a reference (Figures 1 and 3A). To diagnose the FI according to the modified vertical subclassification, the examiners were also asked to measure the length of the shorter root bounding the furcation (which was pre-determined as part of the gold standard assessment) (Figure 3B). All data were recorded on a data collection form in Microsoft Excel(Excel 2016 Inc, Redmond, Washington, USA).

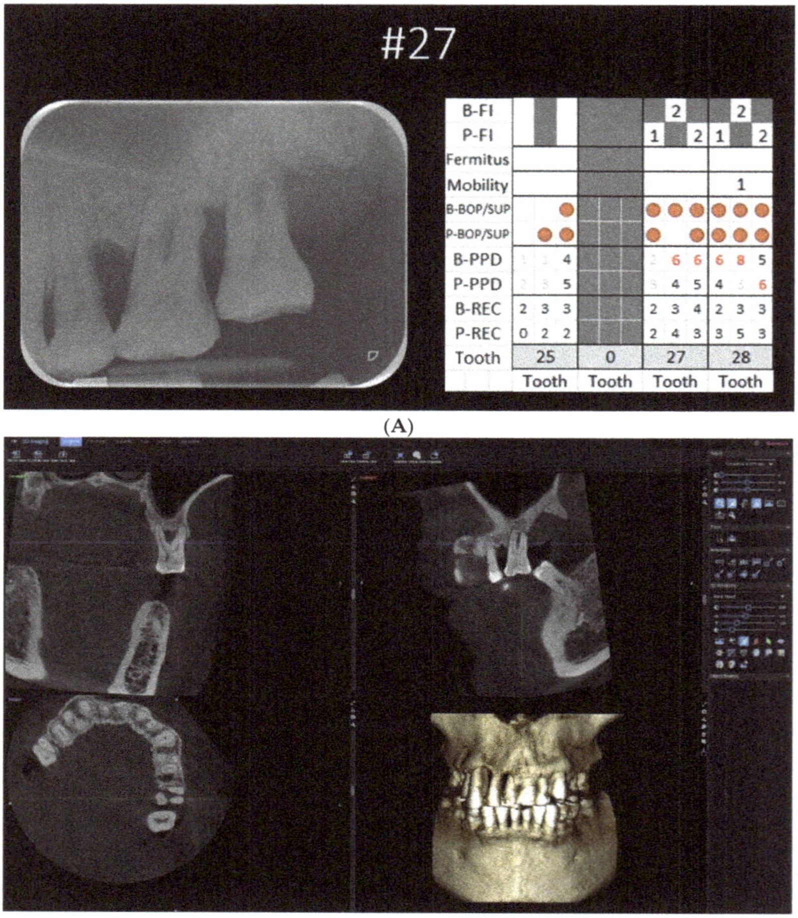

Figure 1. (**A**) Case example with a complete set of clinical periodontal record, periapical radiograph, and CBCT DICOM files as viewed on Romexis Viewer (Planmeca). (**B**) The CBCT viewer axis was first aligned along the long axis of the tooth at the sagittal section and coronal section. At the axial section, the sagittal and coronal planes were adjusted to intersect the canal orifices of the two roots bounding the concerned furcation involvement.

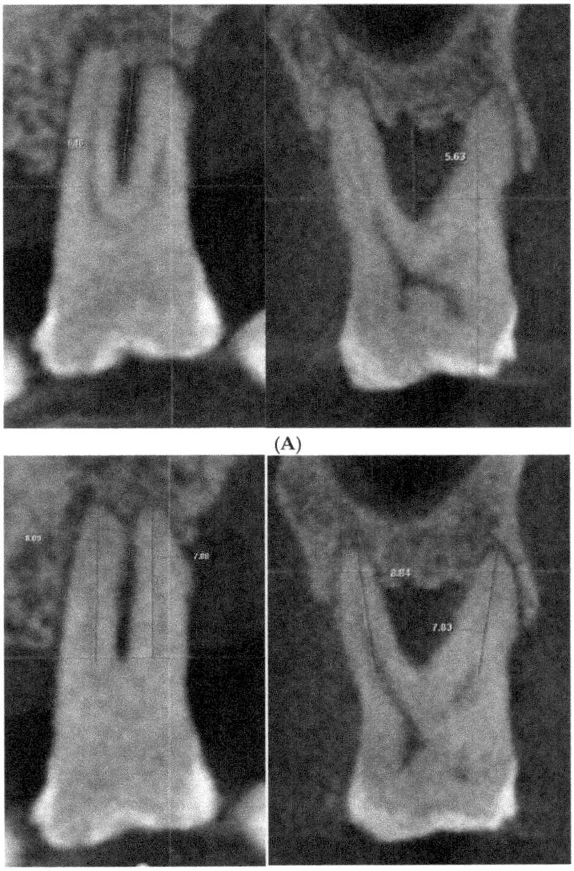

(A)

(B)

Figure 2. (**A**) Measurement of vertical depth of furcation and root length on Romexis (Planmeca). (**B**) By toggling the CBCT along the adjusted axis, the maximal vertical distance from the furcation fornix to the base of the defect and the length of the shorter root bounding the furcation were measured.

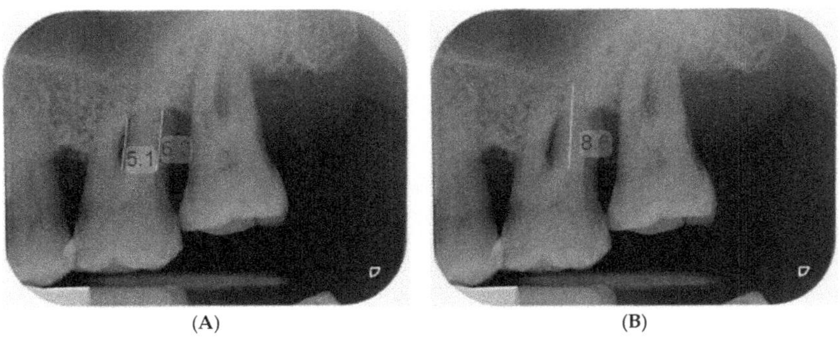

(A) (B)

Figure 3. Measurement of vertical depth of furcation (**A**) and root length (**B**) on periapical radiograph using the measuring tool of Romexis (Planmeca).

2.6. Statistical Analysis

The data collection form in Microsoft Excel was proofed for entry error and inputted into the statistical program SPSS 28.0 (IBM, Armonk, NY, USA) for statistical analysis. The significance of differences in the depth of vertical furcal bone loss between the conventional modality measurement and the gold standard of each examiner was computed with ICC for (i) all 40 teeth, (ii) maxillary molars, and (iii) mandibular molars. Similarly, the significance of differences in the vertical furcation subclassification determined using the conventional modality against the gold standard of each examiner was computed with LWK. The reliability of the conventional modality in determining the vertical depth of furcation involvement and vertical subclassification among the 15 examiners was calculated using the ICC and Fleiss' multirater kappa. All 40 teeth were included and subdivided according to the tooth position (maxillary/mandibular) and the horizontal furcation involvement distribution.

The ICC and Fleiss' kappa between the subgroups were compared using the *F*-test and *Z*-test, respectively, at a significance level of 0.05.

To explore if tooth position (maxillary/mandibular), FI distribution, and examiner experience level affect the bias in measuring the vertical depth of FI, a linear mixed model considering both random intercept and repeated measurements by raters on 40 teeth was performed.

3. Results

Among the 40 selected subject teeth, 20 were maxillary molars, and 20 were mandibular molars. Four maxillary molars had isolated class II horizontal involvement at the buccal furcation. Eight had isolated class II horizontal involvement at either the mesial or distal furcation, and eight had at least two class II or class III horizontal furcation involvements. On the other hand, ten mandibular molars were presented with class II horizontal involvement at either the buccal or lingual furcation, and ten had class II involvement on both sides or class III furcation involvement. When compared against the gold standard vertical depth as measured on CBCT, the 15 examiners displayed an intraclass correlation coefficient range of 0.133–0.570. A higher ICC value could be observed in mandibular molars analysed individually, although statistical significance was only reached in the *F*-test analysis from 5 of the 15 examiners (Table 1). When vertical subclassification assignment was compared against CBCT, the examiners displayed an LWK range of 0.071–0.350. Similarly, when maxillary and mandibular molars were analysed individually, a general trend of a higher LWK value could be observed in mandibular molars. However, statistical significance was only reached in the *Z*-test analysis from 5 out of the 15 examiners (Table 2).

Table 1. Intraclass correlation coefficient (ICC) for vertical depth of furcation involvement measured by conventional modality against CBCT.

Level 1 Examiner	**1**	**2**	**3**	**4**	**5**
All Teeth (95% CI)	0.52 (0.258, 0.712)	0.432 (0.142, 0.654)	0.402 (0.120, 0.628)	0.502 (0.234–0.700)	0.570 (0.322, 0.746)
Maxillary Molar (95% CI)	0.382 (−0.068, 0.700)	0.074 (−0.397, 0.499)	0.054 (−0.348, 0.461)	0.329 (−0.141, 0.671)	0.518 (0.131, 0.773)
Mandibular Molar (95% CI)	0.601 (0.213, 0.822)	0.775 (0.520, 0.904)	0.634 (0.290, 0.835)	0.702 (0.274,0.882)	0.559 (0.157, 0.800)
"*p*-value" (*F*-test)	0.174	0.002	0.022	0.042	0.424
Level 2 Examiner	**6**	**7**	**8**	**9**	**10**
All Teeth (95% CI)	0.133 (−0.147, 0.407)	0.331 (0.044, 0.573)	0.255 (−0.025, 0.509)	0.347 (0.039, 0.594)	0.287 (0.002, 0.537)
Upper Molar (95% CI)	−0.207 (−0.594, 0.252)	−0.001 (−0.348, 0.394)	0.382 (−0.019, 0.690)	0.204 (−0.224, 0.578)	0.022 (−0.361, 0.429)
Lower Molar (95% CI)	0.461 (−0.001, 0.754)	0.637 (0.271, 0.840)	0.079 (−0.230, 0.437)	0.523 (0.133, 0.776)	0.536 (0.003, 0.810)
"*p*-value" (*F*-test)	0.0435	0.016	0.196	0.137	0.0563

Table 1. *Cont.*

Level 3 Examiner	11	12	13	14	15
All Teeth (95% CI)	0.293 (−0.025–0.558)	0.442 (0.161, 0.658)	0.518 (0.247, 0.714)	0.352 (0.055, 0.594)	0.509 (0.243, 0.705)
Upper Molar (95% CI)	0.148 (−0.236, 0.522)	0.149 (−0.227, 0.521)	0.314 (−0.154, 0.662)	0.228 (−0.232, 0.603)	0.368 (−0.095, 0.694)
Lower Molar (95% CI)	0.387 (−0.108, 0.735)	0.567 (0.193, 0.800)	0.679 (0.349, 0.859)	0.468 (−0.103, 0.794)	0.619 (0.253, 0.830)
"*p*-value" (*F*-test)	0.240	0.0749	0.053	0.212	0.139

Table 2. Linear weighted kappa for vertical furcation subclassification determined by conventional modality against CBCT.

Level 1 Examiner	1	2	3	4	5
All Teeth (95% CI)	0.286 (0.049, 0.522)	0.308 (0.081, 0.534)	0.271 (0.018, 0.523)	0.214 (−0.026–0.454)	0.289 (0.051, 0.526)
Maxillary Molar (95% CI)	0.154 (−0.133, 0.441)	0.000 (−0.206, 0.206)	0.085 (−0.204, 0.373)	0.028 (−0.274, 0.330)	0.242 (−0.046, 0.531)
Mandibular Molar (95% CI)	0.394 (0.011, 0.799)	0.596 (0.242, 0.950)	0.394 (−0.011, 0.799)	0.394 (−0.011, 0.799)	0.559 (−0.135, 0.707)
"*p*-value" (*Z*-test)	0.342	0.004	0.222	0.154	0.866
Level 2 Examiner	**6**	**7**	**8**	**9**	**10**
All Teeth (95% CI)	0.071 (−0.154, 0.295)	0.315 (0.071, 0.559)	0.107 (−0.113, 0.398)	0.148 (−0.102, 0.594)	0.194 (−0.023, 0.411)
Upper Molar (95% CI)	−0.216 (−0.447, 0.015)	0.177 (−0.108, 0.462)	−0.053 (−0.270, 0.165)	0.058 (−0.251, 0.367)	−0.087 (−0.309, 0.136)
Lower Molar (95% CI)	0.369 (0.018, 0.721)	0.358 (−0.003, 0.719)	0.174 (−0.191, 0.538)	0.192 (−0.239, 0.623)	0.455 (0.114, 0.795)
"*p*-value" (*Z*-test)	0.006	0.444	0.295	0.621	0.009
Level 3 Examiner	**11**	**12**	**13**	**14**	**15**
All Teeth (95% CI)	0.113 (−0.096–0.323)	0.228 (0.017, 0.439)	0.350 (0.117, 0.582)	0.308 (0.091, 0.524)	0.287 (0.033, 0.541)
Upper Molar (95% CI)	−0.111 (−0.389, 0.167)	−0.087 (−0.182, 0.008)	0.179 (−0.109, 0.468)	0.110 (−0.153, 0.372)	0.143 (−0.188, 0.474)
Lower Molar (95% CI)	0.333 (−0.096, 0.571)	0.500 (0.122, 0.878)	0.490 (0.106, 0.874)	0.464 (0.141, 0.788)	0.406 (0.015, 0.797)
"*p*-value" (*Z*-test)	0.017	0.003	0.204	0.096	0.314

The reliability in measuring the vertical depth of FI conventionally among the 15 examiners was also assessed with an ICC value of 0.560 (95% CI 0.446–0.686), thus suggesting a fair agreement between the examiners [18]. A similar agreement was also found when maxillary and mandibular molars were considered separately, with an ICC value of 0.497 (95% CI 0.343–0.689) and 0.573 (95% CI 0.415–0.750), respectively. No statistical significance was found when the two ICC values were compared ($p = 0.362$). Interestingly when maxillary molars were assessed according to their FI topography, ICC values varied between 0.491 (95% CI 0.199–0.934) for isolated buccal class II FI, 0.470 (95% CI 0.250–0.796) for isolated mesial or distal class II FI, and 0.624 (95% CI 0.395–0.877) in the case of two class II or class III FIs. As for the mandibular molars, ICC values of 0.544 (95% CI 0.334–0.807) in the case of isolated buccal/lingual class II FI and 0.505 (95% CI 0.297–0.783) for buccal and lingual class II or class III FI were found. No statistically significant difference was found under *F*-test analysis for all subgroups in both the upper and lower molars (Table 3).

Table 3. Intraclass correlation coefficient (ICC) for assessment of reliability among the 15 examiners using the conventional modality in measuring vertical depth of furcation.

All Teeth (95% CI)	0.560 (0.446, 0.686)
Maxillary Molar (95% CI)	0.497 (0.343, 0.689)
Mandibular Molar (95% CI)	0.573 (0.415, 0.750)
Isolated Class II at B(Buccal) (95% CI)	0.491 (0.199, 0.934)
Isolated Class II at M/D(mesio/distal) (95% CI)	0.470 (0.250, 0.796)
At Least 2 Class II/Class III (95% CI)	0.624 (0.395, 0.877)
Isolated Class II at B/L(bucco/lingual) (95% CI)	0.544 (0.334, 0.807)
Class II at B/L or Class III (95% CI)	0.505 (0.297, 0.783)

(1) The p-value of the F-test analysis between the maxillary molars and mandibular molars was 0.362. (2) In maxillary molars, the p-value of the F-test analysis between the isolated buccal class II furcation group and isolated mesial/distal class II furcation group was 0.537. (3) In maxillary molars, the p-value of the F-test analysis between the isolated mesial/distal class II furcation group and 2 class II furcation/class III furcation group was 0.331. (4) In maxillary molars, the p-value of the F-test analysis between the isolated buccal class II furcation group and 2 class II furcation/class III furcation group was 0.333. (5) In mandibular molars, the p-value of the F-test analysis between the isolated buccal/lingual class II furcation group and 2 class II furcation/class III furcation group was 0.452.

The reliability of the conventional assessment of subclass vertical subclassification among the 15 examiners was assessed with a Fleiss kappa value of 0.452 (95% CI 0.428–0.477), suggesting a moderate agreement between the examiners [19]. When maxillary and mandibular molars were considered separately, Fleiss kappa values of 0.204 (95% CI 0.172–0.237) and 0.568 (95% CI 0.529–0.608) were found, suggesting a fair agreement when diagnosing maxillary molars and a moderate agreement when diagnosing mandibular molars. The better agreement when diagnosing mandibular molars was statistically significant when the two Fleiss kappa values were compared using the Z-test ($p < 0.001$).

Statistically significantly better agreement among the examiners was found in the maxillary isolated buccal class II furcation involvement subgroup compared to the other two subgroups using the Z-test ($p = 0.004$ and <0.001).

As for the mandibular molars, statistically significantly better agreement among the examiners was found in the subgroup with both buccal and lingual class II or class III FI when compared using the Z-test ($p = 0.014$).

A linear mixed model (LMM) was constructed considering the estimated mean difference in the vertical depth of furcation involvement between the conventional modality and CBCT. Cofactors such as the tooth position (maxillary/mandibular), furcation involvement distribution, and examiner experience level were included in the model (Table 4).

Statistically significantly higher bias was observed in maxillary molars exhibiting isolated buccal class II FI compared to maxillary molars with isolated mesial/distal class II FI using Bonferroni multiple comparisons ($p = 0.016$).

Table 4. The relationship between bias in vertical depth of furcation involvement measurement with tooth position, furcation involvement distribution, and examiner experience in the linear mixed model (unadjusted).

Parameter: Tooth Position	Estimate	95% Confidence Interval		*p*-Value	Pairwise Comparison
		Lower Bound	Upper Bound		
Intercept	−0.408	−0.895	0.079	0.098	
Maxillary molar	0.169	−0.520	0.857	0.623	
Mandibular molar	0				
Parameter: Furcation Involvement Distribution					
Intercept	−0.238	−0.854	0.379	0.439	
				0.022	
Isolated maxillary buccal class II furcation involvement	1.216	0.064	2.369	0.039	
Isolated maxillary mesial/distal class II furcation involvement	−0.792	−1.716	0.132	0.091	
At least two maxillary class II furcation involvements or class III furcation involvement	0.172	−0.752	1.097	0.707	[1] > [2]
Isolated mandibular buccal/lingual class II furcation involvement	−0.341	−1.212	0.531	0.433	
Buccal and lingual class II furcation involvement or class III furcation involvement	0				
Parameter: Examiner Experience Level		**Lower Bound**	**Upper Bound**		
Intercept	−0.405	−0.756	−0.054	0.025	
				<0.01	
Level 1 Examiner Experience (recent graduates with less than one year of postgraduate experience)	0.219	0.086	0.352	0.001	[Level 1] > [Level 2] = [Level 3]
Level 2 Examiner Experience (postgraduate clinicians with at least two years of postgraduate experience)	−0.165	−0.334	0.004	0.055	
Level 3 Examiner Experience (specialist periodontists)	0				

The examiner experience level also appeared to affect the bias in measuring the vertical depth of furcation involvement ($p < 0.01$). It was observed that examiners who were recent graduates with less than one year of postgraduate experience (Level 1) had a significantly higher bias when compared to postgraduate clinicians with at least two years of postgraduate experience (Level 2) ($p < 0.001$) and specialist periodontists (Level 3) ($p = 0.004$), as revealed in the Bonferroni multiple comparisons. No statistically significant difference was found among the Level 2 and Level 3 examiners ($p = 0.166$).

Lastly, a statistically significant difference was detected when descriptive statistics and one-way ANOVA were used to compare the vertical depth of FI in different furcation involvement distribution subgroups as measured on CBCT ($p < 0.001$) (Table 5). The LMM was therefore adjusted and re-analysed, but in the adjusted model (Table 6), no statistically significant difference in bias was observed in maxillary molars and mandibular molars presented with different furcation involvement distributions ($p = 0.228$). The examiner experience level still appeared to affect the bias in measuring the vertical depth of furcation involvement ($p < 0.001$). Bonferroni multiple comparisons revealed a significantly higher bias in examiners with Level 1 experience compared to the more experienced Level 2 and 3 examiners ($p < 0.001$ and $p = 0.03$, respectively). No significant difference was observed between Level 2 and 3 examiners ($p = 0.182$).

Table 5. Descriptive statistics and one-way ANOVA comparing the vertical depth of furcation involvement in different furcation involvement distribution subgroups as measured on CBCT.

	N	Mean (mm)	Std. Deviation	Minimum	Maximum	p-Value
Furcation Distribution						<0.001
Isolated maxillary buccal class II furcation involvement	4	4.5475	1.26800	3.06	6.10	
Isolated maxillary mesial/distal class II furcation involvement	8	2.5675	0.82794	1.58	3.81	
At least two maxillary class II furcation involvements or class III furcation involvement	8	3.6463	1.42269	1.61	6.19	
Isolated mandibular buccal/lingual class II furcation involvement	10	1.9250	0.57161	1.24	3.00	
Mandibular buccal and lingual class II furcation involvement or class III furcation involvement	10	3.1480	0.61387	2.08	4.13	
Total	40	2.9658	1.20115	1.24	6.19	

Table 6. The relationship between bias in vertical depth of furcation involvement measurement, furcation involvement distribution, and examiner experience level in the linear mixed model (adjusted for gold standard vertical depth of furcation involvement).

Parameter	Estimate	95% Confidence Interval		p-Value	Bonferroni Multiple Comparisons
		Lower Bound	Upper Bound		
Intercept	−2.117	−3.200	−1.034	<.001	
Furcation Involvement Distribution				0.228	
Isolated maxillary buccal class II furcation involvement	0.399	−0.664	1.461	0.451	
Isolated maxillary mesial/distal class II furcation involvement	−0.486	−1.287	0.315	0.226	
At least two maxillary class II furcation involvements or class III furcation involvement	−0.116	−0.913	0.680	0.768	
Isolated mandibular buccal/lingual class II furcation involvement	0.358	−0.466	1.182	0.384	
Mandibular buccal and lingual class II furcation involvement or class III furcation involvement	0	.	.	.	
Examiner Experience Level				<0.001	[Level 1] > [Level 2] = [Level 3]
Level 1 Examiner Experience (recent graduates with less than one year of postgraduate experience)	0.225	0.092	0.358	0.001	
Level 2 Examiner Experience (postgraduate clinicians with at least two years of postgraduate experience)	−0.162	−0.331	0.007	0.061	
Level 3 Examiner Experience (specialist periodontists)	0	.	.	.	
Gold Standard Vertical Depth	0.573	0.273	0.874	<0.001	

4. Discussion

There are several risks using conventional clinical and radiographic examination, which could prevent the accurate diagnosis of FI, including gingival tissue consistency, inflammation severity, pressure while probing, probe size, probing angulation, and presence of dental restorations. A recent systematic review showed that CBCT was found to be advantageous and accurate in cases of infra-bony defects and FI [20].

In this preliminary study, vertical furcation assessment of 40 molar teeth was performed by 15 examiners using the conventional periodontal diagnostic methods. The agreement in measuring the vertical depth of FI and subclass assignment against CBCT by the 15 examiners was found to be poor to fair. When maxillary and mandibular molars were analysed separately, a general trend of higher ICC and linear weighted kappa values could be observed in mandibular molars. This is partly in agreement with a previous study in which the authors reported a significant difference in the depth of vertical furcal bone loss measured on pre-operative radiographs and intra-surgically in maxillary molars, but not in mandibular molars [21].

During assessment by CBCT, slides showing the maximal vertical furcal bone loss may not constantly occur at the furcation entrance. Intra-surgical measurement theoretically only allows vertical assessment to be conducted at the entrance. It may also be affected by factors such as probe angulation, the position of the furcation entrance, and intra-surgical visibility. Periodontal probes could only provide measurements to the nearest 0.5 mm. This contrasts the measurement tool used in CBCT diagnostic software, in which measurements could be made to the nearest 0.01 mm. This was shown clearly in a retrospective study that concluded that CBCT is validated as a valuable supplemental tool for assessment of molar FI in addition to periodontal probing and intraoral radiographic examinations [22]. Whether CBCT or intra-surgical measurements could better represent the actual vertical furcal bone loss remains a topic to be explored.

Additionally, significantly better agreement in vertical subclass was found among maxillary molars with isolated buccal class II furcation and mandibular molars with both buccal and lingual class II furcation involvement or class III furcation involvement.

A linear mixed model was constructed to explore the relationship between different factors. The model was subsequently adjusted, including the tooth position (maxillary/mandibular), furcation involvement distribution, and examiner experience level. No significant difference in bias was observed between molars of different furcation involvement patterns. Higher bias was observed in examiners with less than one year of postgraduate experience compared to the more experienced clinicians in both the unadjusted and adjusted models. This agrees with a previous study in which a significantly higher horizontal furcation degree assessment accuracy using intraoral radiographs was demonstrated by a more experienced examiner [9].

One major limitation of the current study is the limited sample size. Since 40 molars were included, specific subgroups (maxillary molars with isolated class II buccal furcation involvement) had a much smaller representation when compared to the other subgroups.

Due to the study's retrospective nature, only 6-point periodontal chartings of the subject teeth could be retrieved from the database record; this may not be sufficient to reflect the actual attachment levels around a molar tooth. A difference in attachment levels may exist between the two roots bounding the same furcation, so a clinical assessment of individual roots may provide a better representation.

The current study found poor to fair agreement between the conventional diagnostic modality and CBCT in both the vertical furcal depth and subclassification assignment. Future research may also explore the reliability of using CBCT in the vertical assessment of furcation, and thus a comparison could be performed. Performing a study similar to the current study but with a prospective design and a larger sample size may also increase the power during the analysis.

5. Conclusions

Within the study's limitations, conventional periodontal diagnostic methods based on periapical radiographs and clinical periodontal parameters appear to be in poor to fair agreement with CBCT in measuring the vertical depth of furcation and diagnosing molars according to the modified vertical subclassification. With conventional periodontal diagnostics, fair reliability was found for vertical furcal depth measurement, and moderate reliability was found for vertical subclass assignment. Examiners with the least experience exhibited greater bias when measuring the vertical furcal depth. In summary, it can be suggested that CBCT is beneficial in cases of molars with FI, especially when it comes to surgical treatment planning.

Author Contributions: Conceptualisation, G.P. and J.L.; methodology, G.P. and C.F.; software; validation, J.L. and A.W.K.Y.; formal analysis, J.L.; investigation, M.F.; data curation, G.P. and A.W.K.Y.; writing—original draft preparation, G.P. and J.L.; writing—review and editing, A.A.; visualisation, M.F.; supervision, G.P. All authors have read and agreed to the published version of the manuscript.

Funding: The study was funded by the Periodontal Research Fund of the University of Hong Kong.

Institutional Review Board Statement: The study protocol was approved by the local Institutional Review Board of the University of Hong Kong/Hospital Authority Hong Kong West Cluster (IRB Approval Number: UW22-295 11/05/2022).

Informed Consent Statement: Not applicable.

Data Availability Statement: Not applicable.

Conflicts of Interest: The authors declare no conflict of interest.

References

1. Hamp, S.E.; Nyman, S.; Lindhe, J. Periodontal treatment of multirooted teeth. Results after 5 years. *J. Clin. Periodontol.* **1975**, *2*, 126–135. [CrossRef] [PubMed]
2. Dannewitz, B.; Zeidler, A.; Hüsing, J.; Saure, D.; Pfefferle, T.; Eickholz, P.; Pretzl, B. Loss of molars in periodontally treated patients: Results ten years and more after active periodontal therapy. *J. Clin. Periodontol.* **2016**, *43*, 53–62. [CrossRef] [PubMed]
3. Nibali, L.; Zavattini, A.; Nagata, K.; Di Iorio, A.; Lin, G.-H.; Needleman, I.; Donos, N. Tooth loss in molars with and without furcation involvement—A systematic review and meta-analysis. *J. Clin. Periodontol.* **2016**, *43*, 156–166. [CrossRef] [PubMed]
4. Tarnow, D.; Fletcher, P. Classification of the vertical component of furcation involvement. *J. Periodontol.* **1984**, *55*, 283–284. [CrossRef]
5. Tonetti, M.S.; Christiansen, A.L.; Cortellini, P. Vertical subclassification predicts survival of molars with class II furcation involvement during supportive periodontal care. *J. Clin. Periodontol.* **2017**, *44*, 1140–1144. [CrossRef]
6. Nibali, L.; Sun, C.; Akcalı, A.; Yeh, Y.-C.; Tu, Y.-K.; Donos, N. The effect of horizontal and vertical furcation involvement on molar survival: A retrospective study. *J. Clin. Periodontol.* **2017**, *45*, 373–381. [CrossRef]
7. Cortellini, P.; Cortellini, S.; Tonetti, M.S. Papilla preservation flaps for periodontal regeneration of molars severely compromised by combined furcation and intrabony defects: Retrospective analysis of a registry-based cohort. *J. Periodontol.* **2019**, *91*, 165–173. [CrossRef] [PubMed]
8. Mealey, B.L.; Neubauer, M.F.; Butzin, C.A.; Waldrop, T.C. Use of furcal bone sounding to improve accuracy of furcation diagnosis. *J. Periodontol.* **1994**, *65*, 649–657. [CrossRef]
9. Graetz, C.; Plaumann, A.; Wiebe, J.-F.; Springer, C.; Sälzer, S.; Dörfer, C.E. Periodontal Probing Versus Radiographs for the Diagnosis of Furcation Involvement. *J. Periodontol.* **2014**, *85*, 1371–1379. [CrossRef]
10. Deas, E.; Moritz, A.J.; Mealey, B.L.; McDonnell, H.T.; Powell, C.A. Clinical Reliability of the "Furcation Arrow" as a Diagnostic Marker. *J. Periodontol.* **2006**, *77*, 1436–1441. [CrossRef]
11. Fuhrmann, R.A.W.; Bucker, A.; Diedrich, P.R. Furcation involvement: Comparison of dental radiographs and HR-CT-slices in human specimens. *J. Periodontal Res.* **1997**, *32*, 409–418. [CrossRef] [PubMed]
12. Qiao, J.; Wang, S.; Duan, J.; Zhang, Y.; Qiu, Y.; Sun, C.; Liu, D. The accuracy of cone-beam computed tomography in assessing maxillary molar furcation involvement. *J. Clin. Periodontol.* **2013**, *41*, 269–274. [CrossRef] [PubMed]
13. Feijo, C.V.; De Lucena, J.G.F.; Kurita, L.M.; Pereira, S.L.S. Evaluation of cone beam computed tomography in the detection of horizontal periodontal bone defects: An in vivo study. *Int. J. Periodontics Restor. Dent.* **2012**, *32*, e162–e168.
14. Walter, C.; Kaner, D.; Berndt, D.C.; Weiger, R.; Zitzmann, N.U. Three-dimensional imaging as a pre-operative tool in decision making for furcation surgery. *J. Clin. Periodontol.* **2009**, *36*, 250–257. [CrossRef] [PubMed]
15. Walter, C.; Schmidt, J.C.; Rinne, C.A.; Mendes, S.; Dula, K.; Sculean, A. Cone beam computed tomography (CBCT) for diagnosis and treatment planning in periodontology: Systematic review update. *Clin. Oral Investig.* **2020**, *24*, 2943–2958. [CrossRef]

16. Jolivet, G.; Huck, O.; Petit, C. Evaluation of furcation involvement with diagnostic imaging methods: A systematic review. *Dentomaxillofac. Radiol.* **2022**, *51*, 8. [CrossRef]
17. Yeung, A.W.K.; Jacobs, R.; Bornstein, M.M. Novel low-dose protocols using cone beam computed tomography in dental medicine: A review focusing on indications, limitations, and future possibilities. *Clin. Oral Investig.* **2019**, *23*, 2573–2581. [CrossRef]
18. Cicchetti, D.V.; A Sparrow, S. Developing criteria for establishing interrater reliability of specific items: Applications to assessment of adaptive behavior. *Am. J. Ment. Defic.* **1981**, *86*, 127–137.
19. Altman, D.G. *Practical Statistics for Medical Research*; Chapman & Hall: New York, NY, USA, 1990; pp. 132–146. [CrossRef]
20. Assiri, H.; Dawasaz, A.A.; AlAhmari, A.; Asiri, Z. Cone beam computed tomography (CBCT) in periodontal diseases: A Systematic review based on the efficacy model. *BMC Oral Health* **2020**, *20*, 191. [CrossRef]
21. Yusof, N.A.M.; Noor, E.; Reduwan, N.H.; Yusof, M.Y.P.M. Diagnostic accuracy of periapical radiograph, cone beam computed tomography, and intrasurgical linear measurement techniques for assessing furcation defects: A longitudinal randomised controlled trial. *Clin. Oral Investig.* **2020**, *25*, 923–932. [CrossRef]
22. Zhang, W.; Foss, K.; Wang, B.Y. A retrospective study on molar furcation assessment via clinical detection, intraoral radiography and cone beam computed tomography. *BMC Oral Health* **2018**, *18*, 75. [CrossRef]

Disclaimer/Publisher's Note: The statements, opinions and data contained in all publications are solely those of the individual author(s) and contributor(s) and not of MDPI and/or the editor(s). MDPI and/or the editor(s) disclaim responsibility for any injury to people or property resulting from any ideas, methods, instructions or products referred to in the content.

diagnostics

MDPI

Review

Current Applications of Deep Learning and Radiomics on CT and CBCT for Maxillofacial Diseases

Kuo Feng Hung [1], Qi Yong H. Ai [2], Lun M. Wong [3], Andy Wai Kan Yeung [4], Dion Tik Shun Li [1] and Yiu Yan Leung [1,*]

1 Oral and Maxillofacial Surgery, Faculty of Dentistry, The University of Hong Kong, Hong Kong SAR, China
2 Health Technology and Informatics, The Hong Kong Polytechnic University, Hong Kong SAR, China
3 Imaging and Interventional Radiology, Faculty of Medicine, The Chinese University of Hong Kong, Hong Kong SAR, China
4 Oral and Maxillofacial Radiology, Applied Oral Sciences and Community Dental Care, Faculty of Dentistry, The University of Hong Kong, Hong Kong SAR, China
* Correspondence: myyleung@hku.hk

Abstract: The increasing use of computed tomography (CT) and cone beam computed tomography (CBCT) in oral and maxillofacial imaging has driven the development of deep learning and radiomics applications to assist clinicians in early diagnosis, accurate prognosis prediction, and efficient treatment planning of maxillofacial diseases. This narrative review aimed to provide an up-to-date overview of the current applications of deep learning and radiomics on CT and CBCT for the diagnosis and management of maxillofacial diseases. Based on current evidence, a wide range of deep learning models on CT/CBCT images have been developed for automatic diagnosis, segmentation, and classification of jaw cysts and tumors, cervical lymph node metastasis, salivary gland diseases, temporomandibular (TMJ) disorders, maxillary sinus pathologies, mandibular fractures, and dentomaxillofacial deformities, while CT-/CBCT-derived radiomics applications mainly focused on occult lymph node metastasis in patients with oral cancer, malignant salivary gland tumors, and TMJ osteoarthritis. Most of these models showed high performance, and some of them even outperformed human experts. The models with performance on par with human experts have the potential to serve as clinically practicable tools to achieve the earliest possible diagnosis and treatment, leading to a more precise and personalized approach for the management of maxillofacial diseases. Challenges and issues, including the lack of the generalizability and explainability of deep learning models and the uncertainty in the reproducibility and stability of radiomic features, should be overcome to gain the trust of patients, providers, and healthcare organizers for daily clinical use of these models.

Keywords: artificial intelligence; deep learning; radiomics; computed tomography; cone-beam computed tomography; maxillofacial diseases

1. Introduction

Technological advances are changing many aspects of our society and industries, including healthcare. Innovative digital technologies such as computer-aided design/manufacturing, rapid prototyping, augmented/virtual reality, and "omics" analysis have been increasingly used in several medical and dental disciplines for diagnostic and therapeutic purposes [1]. Artificial intelligence (AI) is one of the most innovative and disruptive technologies that has the potential to revolutionize current clinical practice and research. The concept of AI was coined in the 1950s, referring to the idea of building machines that can imitate human behavior to perform complex tasks [2]. Since the 1950s, there were two "AI winters" in the 1970s and late 1980s, which occurred mainly due to insufficient computational power and resources, leading to a huge gap between the expectations and the actual outcomes of AI models of the time (i.e., knowledge-based expert systems) [2,3]. In the late 2000s, the advent of advanced graphics processing units reignited the enthusiasm for the development of various AI technologies and applications, such as intelligent robotics, autonomous vehicles, machine learning, computer vision, and natural language processing (Figure 1) [4].

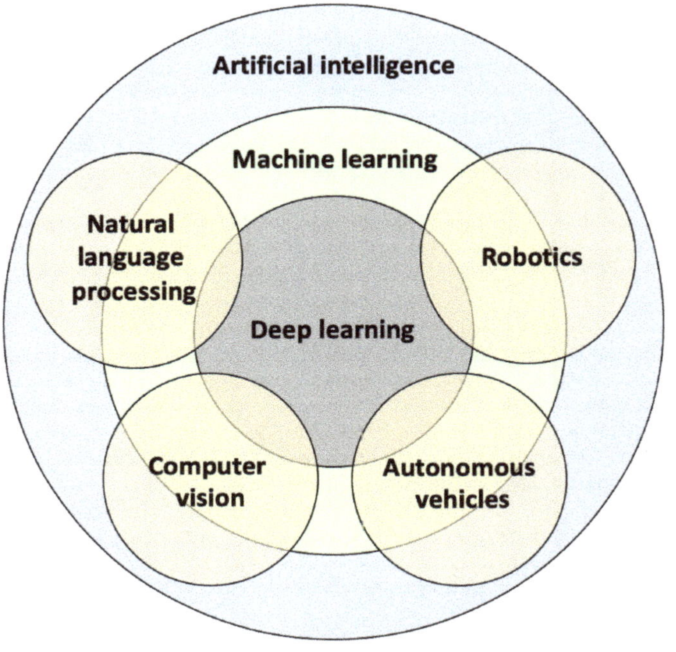

Figure 1. Artificial intelligence and its subfields.

Machine learning is a subfield of AI that enables algorithms to learn the intrinsic statistical patterns in a set of data without being explicitly programmed and then to make predictions on unseen data [2]. Due to the characteristics of data (e.g., clinical, biological, and radiographic data) and the major problems left unsolved in medicine and dentistry (e.g., early diagnosis, accurate prediction, and efficient treatment of specific diseases), machine learning and its subset deep learning are the most widely employed techniques in these fields [3]. Deep learning, a subset of machine learning, specifically uses multi-layered artificial neural networks to learn representations of data with multiple levels of abstraction [5]. Deep learning algorithms are trained to automatically extract hierarchical features in complex data and optimize the weighted parameters, leading to a more efficient learning process and minimized prediction errors. Within deep learning, the convolutional neural network (CNN) is a class of artificial neural networks that has been frequently used for image-related tasks, such as automated detection, segmentation, and classification of complex patterns in two-dimensional (2D) and three-dimensional (3D) images [3].

Radiomics is an emerging translational field in quantitative imaging, related to machine learning. It is capable of quantifying the textural information of specific regions of interest in digital diagnostic images through mathematic extraction of signal intensity distribution and pixel/voxel interrelationships that cannot be perceived by the human eye [6]. Based on high-throughput analysis of quantitative imaging features for the characterization of tissues, radiomics applications, similar to other omics clusters (e.g., genomics, proteomics, and metabolomics), have the potential to promote personalized diagnosis and management of interested diseases or conditions [5]. Currently, a wide range of radiomics models have been developed in many medical fields to assist clinicians in the screening, diagnosis, risk stratification, treatment response monitoring, and outcome prediction of malignancies, such as nasopharyngeal, lung, and breast cancer [6–8]. In general, AI and radiomics are interconnected and mutually reinforcing. AI, particularly machine learning, can serve as a powerful data modeling tool to analyze a massive number of radiomic features and parameters, while interpretation of radiomic features may provide information to better understand the decision-making process of a trained AI model.

Radiographic examination is an integral component in the diagnosis and management of most dento-maxillofacial diseases, and so a great amount of digital radiographic images are readily available in the archiving systems and associated databases of many hospitals and clinics. Hence, the majority of AI models in dentistry have been developed based on radiographic images to assist dentists in the diagnosis (e.g., detection of a certain pathology), treatment planning (e.g., segmentation of anatomical structures and pathologies), and prediction (e.g., classification of individuals with a higher possibility of good/poor treatment outcome) of various dental and maxillofacial diseases [3]. Computed tomography (CT) and cone-beam computed tomography (CBCT) are the most common 3D imaging modalities used in many dental specialties, especially in oral and maxillofacial surgery. Compared with conventional 2D dental radiography (i.e., periapical, bitewing, panoramic, and cephalometric radiography), CT/CBCT allows for the visualization of anatomical structures and pathologies in 3D, thus capable of providing not only higher diagnostic accuracy but also more detailed information regarding the true morphology, volume, and location of the lesions. As CBCT has gained increasing popularity in daily dental practice, this imaging modality is considered as an ideal data source for developing clinically practicable AI tools to improve the accuracy and efficiency of the diagnosis and treatment of maxillofacial diseases [9]. According to a recent systematic review, the number of AI models developed on CBCT images for dento-maxillofacial applications has increased dramatically over the years since the mid-2010s, particularly using deep learning [10]. Therefore, this narrative review aimed to provide an up-to-date overview of the current applications of deep learning and radiomics on CT and CBCT for the diagnosis and management of maxillofacial diseases.

2. Deep Learning and Radiomics on CT/CBCT for the Diagnosis and Management of Maxillofacial Diseases

Maxillofacial diseases include both odontogenic and nonodontogenic diseases in the jaws and related structures including salivary glands, temporomandibular joints (TMJs), and facial muscles. Due to their anatomical complexity and proximity to critical vascular and neural structures, 3D imaging (such as CT/CBCT) is often required in the diagnostic and treatment planning processes, serving as one of the essential components of digital workflows for patient management. Thus, a wide range of deep learning and radiomics applications have been developed based on CT/CBCT images for diagnosis, treatment planning, and prediction of various maxillofacial diseases (Tables 1 and 2).

2.1. *Jaw Cysts and Tumors*

Incidental findings of lesions in the jaws are often observed on routine dental radiographic examination. These lesions are usually cystic in nature and thus challenging for general practitioners to differentiate between cysts and tumors on radiographic images. Motivated by the need for more timely and accurate diagnosis of maxillofacial cysts and tumors, several studies have developed AI, especially deep learning, models on 2D panoramic radiographs for automatic diagnosis of various cysts and tumors of the jaws [11–15]. Most of them focused on the lesions including ameloblastoma, odontogenic keratocysts (OKCs), dentigerous cysts, radicular cysts, and bone cysts, and the proposed models obtained high diagnostic accuracy on par with oral–maxillofacial surgeons.

Differentiating various types of jaw cysts and tumors on CBCT using deep learning has been proposed by several groups [16–18]. Lee et al. developed CNN models for automatic detection, segmentation, and classification of OKCs, dentigerous and periapical cysts on panoramic and CBCT images [16]. Not surprisingly, the model trained on CBCT images outperformed the one on panoramic radiographs, which may result from the advantages of CBCT in depicting the lesion morphology in 3D with more quantitative features in each voxel of the lesion region. Bispo et al. [17] and Chai et al. [18] developed CNN models to automatically classify between ameloblastoma and OKCs on CT images, respectively. Chai et al. compared the model's performance with seven senior and thirty junior oral–maxillofacial surgeons. The model outperformed both senior and junior oral-maxillofacial surgeons with an accuracy of 85% in a short execution time of nearly 3 milliseconds per scan. These deep learning models have the potential to assist general dental practitioners in identifying different types of jaw cysts and tumors on CBCT images during daily dental practice, which would facilitate timely referral to oral–maxillofacial specialists and thus allow for the earliest possible treatment.

2.2. Lymph Node Metastasis

Oral squamous cell carcinoma (OSCC) is the sixth most frequent malignancy globally and associated with a high rate of invasiveness and lymph node metastasis [19]. Cervical lymph node metastasis has been reported as one of the major prognostic factors in OSCC patients that is directly correlated with a reduced overall survival rate. Patients with OSCC routinely have prophylactic neck dissection, as occult lymph node metastasis is not uncommon in clinical practice [20]. However, the neck dissection may result in severe functional and sensory complications (such as accessory or facial nerve paralysis and stiffness of the shoulder and neck), which considerably influence the patients' quality of life [20]. Therefore, the controversy in the prophylactic neck dissection for patients with OSCC drives the search in non-invasive approaches with high accuracy in identifying lymph node metastasis. Contrast-enhanced CT is one of the most common imaging modalities used for the diagnosis of lymph node metastasis in OSCC patients. Size, necrosis, and extranodal extension are the main features for identifying cervical lymph node metastasis. However, complete detection of all metastatic lymph nodes using CT images based only on the perceivable nodal features is still challenging [21]. AI seems to be able to promote the development of a non-invasive approach for accurate identification of the nature of cervical lymph nodes in patients with OSCC.

Ariji et al. first developed a CNN model to differentiate histopathologically proven metastatic cervical lymph nodes from the negative ones on cropped contrast-enhanced CT images of OSCC patients [22]. The model achieved favorable accuracy with an AUC (area under the curve) of 0.80, which is similar to the level of two experienced radiologists (AUC of 0.83). Subsequently, Ariji et al. further proposed a CNN model to differentiate between metastatic lymph nodes with and without extranodal extension on cropped contrast-enhanced CT images of OSCC patients [23]. The model achieved high accuracy with an AUC of 0.82 and outperformed four experienced radiologists (AUCs of 0.52–0.63). However, these models could only make decisions on the cropped images of individual lymph nodes so that manual identification and cropping of all cervical lymph nodes on multiple CT image slices were required. Manual identification and cropping works are time-consuming, which would probably limit the implementation of these models for routine clinical use. In order to improve their clinical applicability, Ariji et al. developed CNN models for automated detection and segmentation of metastatic and non-metastatic cervical lymph nodes on contrast-enhanced CT images [24,25]. The latest model (AUC of 0.95) outperformed two experienced radiologists (AUC of 0.90) in detecting metastatic cervical lymph nodes while its segmentation accuracy should be further improved.

The potential of radiomics in the screening, diagnosis, and prediction of oral, head and neck cancer has been increasingly exploited [5]. Few studies investigated whether radiomic features extracted from CT/CBCT images could be used for predictive analysis of lymph node metastasis in patients with oral, head and neck cancer (Table 2). Kubo et al. developed predictive models based on CT-derived radiomic features using various machine learning classifiers for occult cervical lymph node metastasis in patients with tongue cancer [26]. The model trained with support vector machine (SVM) obtained the highest accuracy in predicting regional lymph node metastasis with an AUC of 0.98. Zhong et al. developed predictive models based on CT-derived radiomic features and associated clinical parameters for occult cervical lymph node metastasis in patients with tongue cancer [27]. The model on radiomic features and clinical lymph node status achieved higher prediction accuracy (AUC of 0.94) than the one only on radiomic features (AUC of 0.92). Morgan et al. developed several models based on CT- and CBCT-derived radiomic features and/or several clinical parameters using an explainable boosting machine for predicting local failure in head and neck cancer [28]. The model trained on both radiomic features and clinical parameters achieved the highest predictive performance with an AUC of 0.87 for primary cancer and 0.91 for nodal structures. The use of these models may enable a more personalized management of patients with oral, head and neck cancer.

2.3. Salivary Gland Diseases

Salivary gland diseases are a group of inflammatory, infectious, and neoplastic conditions, mainly occurring in the parotid glands, followed by minor salivary glands, submandibular glands, and sublingual glands. Diagnosis of salivary gland diseases is a great challenge in dentistry and oto-rhino-laryngology, as it heavily relies on the practitioners' experiences and diagnostic imaging. Deep learning models for the diagnosis of salivary gland diseases have been developed largely on magnetic resonance imaging (MRI) scans [29] because of its advantages over other imaging modalities in depicting soft tissues. Nevertheless, MRI is not widely available in healthcare settings, and thus, CT remains an important role in identifying and describing the extent of neoplasms. Applying deep learning to CT images may expand its scope in the diagnosis of salivary gland diseases. Kise et al. developed a CNN model on CT images to automatically detect the fatty degeneration of the salivary gland that is a key characteristic finding for the diagnosis of Sjogren's syndrome [30]. The model performed similarly to three experienced radiologists and outperformed three inexperienced radiologists. Additionally, deep learning models on CT achieved promising performance in differentiating various types of salivary gland tumors. Yuan et al. developed a CNN model to classify between pleomorphic adenoma and malignant parotid gland tumors on CT images [31]. The model achieved high classification accuracy of 90%. Zhang et al. trained several CNN models for classification between benign and malignant parotid gland tumors on CT images [32]. The customized CNN model achieved the highest classification accuracy of up to 98% as compared with the models built based on the pre-trained CNNs, including VGG16, InceptionV3, ResNet, and DenseNet.

The intrinsic radiomic features of malignant parotid gland tumors on CT images may be extracted to assist in differentiating between benign and malignant salivary gland tumors (Table 2). Zhang et al. developed a multivariable logistic regression model based on CT-derived radiomic features to classify between low- and high-grade mucoepidermoid carcinoma of the salivary glands [33]. The model showed that high-grade mucoepidermoid carcinomas may be associated with low energy, high correlation texture, and high surface irregularity. Xu et al. developed predictive models based on individual or combined CT-derived radiomic features and radiological variables (i.e., the location and metastases of lymph nodes) to differentiate between benign and malignant parotid gland tumors [34]. The model trained using SVM on CT-derived radiomic features and the location and metastases of lymph nodes achieved the highest performance than the models on individual radiomic features or radiological variables. Liu et al. developed predictive models based on either MRI or CT-derived radiomic features for differentiating between pleomorphic adenoma and Warthin tumors of the parotid glands, respectively [35]. The model on MRI-derived radiomic features (AUC of 0.91) performed slightly higher than but not significantly different from the model on CT-derived radiomic features (AUC of 0.88). These models may serve as auxiliary tools to assist clinicians in identifying patients with malignant salivary gland tumors.

2.4. Temporomandibular Joint Disorders

TMJ disorders are one of the most common orofacial dysfunctions that frequently cause joint clicking sounds, limited mouth opening, pain, and headache [36]. Degenerative bony changes is one of the main causes associated with TMJ disorders, which may start with the flattening or sclerosis of the mandibular condyle head, followed by the erosion of its cortical surface, and eventually osteoarthritis [37]. Accurate diagnosis of TMJ disorders is difficult for general dental practitioners and requires adequate clinical experience to avoid patients undergoing unnecessary examinations and invasive treatment. CBCT imaging is commonly used for assessing the morphology of TMJs. However, a low consistency among clinicians was found in the subjective interpretation of morphological changes in the TMJs [37], indicating that a quantitative diagnostic tool for TMJ disorders would be of great clinical value. Le et al. developed a CNN model for automated segmentation of the mandibular ramus and condyle on CBCT images [38]. Kim et al. developed a CNN model to automatically segment and measure the cortical thickness of the mandibular condyle head on CBCT images [39]. The model achieved favorable performance with a short execution time of nearly 10 s, which may contribute to automated quantitative analysis of the changes in bony structures of TMJs. de Dumast et al. developed a deep learning model on CBCT images to classify the morphological variations of TMJ osteoarthritis into five categories [40]. The model achieved high classification agreement of 91% with two human experts, demonstrating its potential to assist clinicians in the diagnosis of TMJ osteoarthritis. Bianchi et al. developed diagnostic models based on radiomic, biomolecular, clinical, and demographic features using different machine learning algorithms for TMJ osteoarthritis [41]. The model trained using the combination of XGBoost (Extreme Gradient Boosting) and LightGBM (Light Gradient Boosting Machine) algorithms achieved the highest accuracy with an AUC of 0.82. With the aid of this diagnostic model, screening individuals with early TMJ osteoarthritis seems possible.

2.5. Maxillary Sinus Pathologies

The maxillary sinus is the largest paranasal sinus and is frequently involved in various dento-maxillofacial surgical procedures, such as apical surgeries of the maxillary posterior teeth and sinus augmentation for dental implant placement [42,43]. Accurate diagnosis and classification of maxillary sinus pathologies prior to surgical procedures involving the sinus region is one of the key factors to ensure a predictable treatment outcome [44,45]. However, general practitioners may be less confident in diagnosing maxillary sinus pathologies on radiographic images due to their unfamiliarity with the anatomical structures and pathologies of the sinus. Implementation of dento-maxillofacial surgical procedures in the maxillary sinus with pathological changes are very likely to increase the risk of ostiomeatal dysfunction and sinus infection [46]. Some deep learning models on 2D radiographic images achieved favorable performance in detecting maxillary sinus pathologies [3]. One of the main limitations of the models on 2D images is their inculpability of providing information regarding the true morphology, volume, and location of the detected lesions, which are important in the planning of an appropriate treatment strategy for surgical procedures in the sinus region. Currently, CNN models were developed for automated segmentation of the maxillary sinus [47,48] and the morphological changes of the sinus mucosa [49,50] on CT/CBCT images. Jung et al. developed a CNN model on CBCT images to segment maxillary sinus pathologies including the mucosal thickening and mucous retention cysts of the sinus [49]. The model obtained favorable segmentation performance on internal data while its performance was inferior on external images. The scans including the maxillary sinus are frequently taken with a large field of view (FOV) and thus are associated with higher radiation exposure to the patients [51]. The use of a low-dose imaging protocol has been strongly recommended for large FOV scans of the sinus [52]. Hung et al. reported that their 3D CNN model achieved high performance on both standard-dose (AUCs of 0.89–0.93) and low-dose (AUCs of 0.84–0.89) CBCT images in automatic detection, segmentation, and measurement of the mucosal thickening and mucous retention cysts of the sinus [50]. No significant differences were found in the volume of the sinus, the lesions, and their ratio between automated and manual measurements. This CNN model has the potential to assist clinicians in identifying maxillary sinus lesions, evaluating the extent of sinus opacification, and planning surgical procedures in the sinus region.

2.6. Mandibular Fractures

The mandible is the only moveable and the most commonly fractured bone of the face in trauma cases. A CNN model was developed to automatically detect mandibular fractures on CT images [53]. The models first generated a synthesized panoramic image from the original CT scan. The mandibular region in the synthesized panoramic image was subsequently straightened and divided into image patches of nine subregions, including symphysis, left/right parasymphysis, left/right mandibular body, left/right mandibular angle, and left/right condylar process. Eventually, the model determined the presence or absence of a fracture on the image patches of specific mandibular subregions. This model achieved high fracture detection accuracy with AUC values of 0.93–0.98 across the nine mandibular subregions, which may be particularly useful for detecting occult condylar fractures.

2.7. Dentofacial Deformities and Malocclusion

Dentofacial deformities and malocclusion are characterized by abnormalities of the dentition, jaws, and face that affect not only the oral function and appearance of patients but also their physical, social, and psychological well-being. Orthodontic and orthognathic treatment is commonly performed to correct these abnormalities. Conventional treatment planning of orthognathic surgery consists of a series of steps based on clinical examination, cephalometric analysis, dental casts, facebow, and articulators. Compared with the conventional approach, a digital workflow improves the accuracy and efficiency of orthognathic surgery without the need of a facebow record and model surgery [54].

The digital workflows in dentistry frequently require a 3D virtual augmented patient model that is created based on multimodal image data (such as CBCT and optical intra-oral, facial, and/or model scans) to serve as the foundation for subsequent treatment planning and guided surgery for many surgical procedures including orthognathic surgery. Segmentation of anatomical structures and multimodal image registration are the essential steps in the process of building a virtual patient model. They can be performed manually through visual inspection or semi-automatically by using the fiducial marker registration method or surface-based matching algorithm [55]. The manual approach is time-consuming, and errors by visual inspection are unavoidable. While the semi-automatic approach can improve the efficiency of these steps, manual correction is still necessary prior to further planning steps, such as the design of surgical splints for orthognathic corrections. Deep learning models for automatically segmenting anatomical structures on CBCT images or merging the contour of the interested region from different image datasets may be a solution to improving the accuracy and efficiency of image segmentation and registration. Commercially available AI platforms, such as CranioCatch (Eskişehir, Turkey), Denti.AI (Toronto, ON, Canada), Diagnocat (Tel Aviv, Israel), Promaton (Amsterdam, The Netherlands), and Relu (Leuven, Belgium), and several CNN models have been proposed for automated segmentation of dento-maxillofacial anatomical structures (including teeth, jaws, maxillary sinus, pharyngeal airway, mandibular canal, palatine, zygomatic, nasal, and lacrimal bones) on CBCT images (Figure 2) [56–63]. Some of them performed similarly to experienced radiologists and outperformed other semi-automatic software, such as Mimics® (version 23.0, Materialise N.V., Leuven, Belgium). Automated multimodal image registration to merge CBCT and optical intra-oral/model scans using deep learning has been proposed by some groups [64,65]. The model by Jang et al. showed high accuracy with a mean registration error of 0.5 mm, which is less than that of the manual registration approach (1.7 mm) [64]. The model by Chung et al. completed the image registration procedure in a short period of nearly 20 s with registration errors less than that of the conventional three-point registration method [65]. The model's performance was not affected by the presence of metal artifacts on CBCT images, which may greatly improve image registration accuracy in patients with multiple metallic dental restorations.

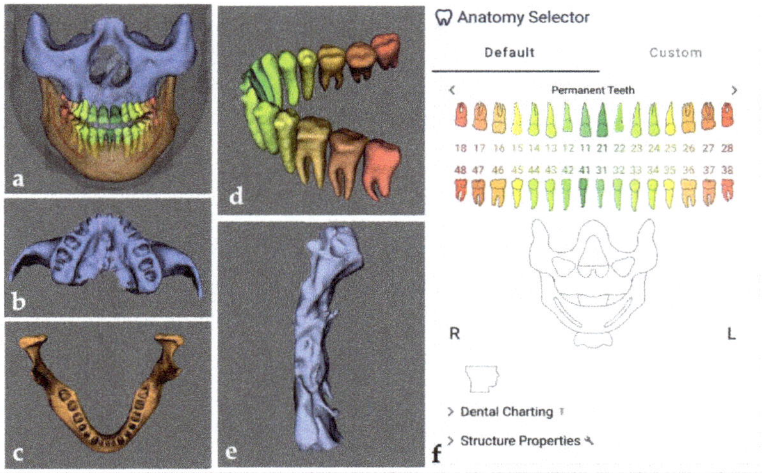

Figure 2. Example of automated segmentation of dento-maxillofacial anatomical structures on CBCT images using a commercially available AI software platform, Relu (Leuven, Belgium; available at https://relu.eu (accessed on 5 December 2022)). The overview of the segmented anatomical structures (**a**), including the maxilla (**b**), mandible (**c**), teeth with orthodontic brackets (**d**), and pharyngeal airway (**e**), and automated labeling of teeth (**f**).

In addition, deep learning was applied to determine whether an individual needs orthognathic surgery and to predict the surgical outcomes. Kim et al. developed several CNN models on CBCT images to automatically classify individuals into Class I, II, and III skeletal malocclusion according to several parameters including the anteroposterior relationship of the maxillary and mandibular first molars and the alignment of teeth with reference to the line of occlusion [66]. The performance of the developed models was up to an accuracy of 93.8%. The model may facilitate orthognathic evaluation by identifying individuals in need of surgical correction of skeletal malocclusion. Few CNN models were developed on CT/CBCT images to predict the changes in the skeletal and soft-tissue profile after orthognathic surgery [67–69]. The model by ter Horst et al. for soft-tissue profile prediction performed similarly to a soft tissue prediction model (mass tensor model) that is widely used for maxillofacial surgical planning [67]. These predictive models may assist surgeons in orthognathic surgical planning to improve postoperative facial symmetry.

Table 1. Performance of deep learning models on CT/CBCT images for the diagnosis and treatment planning of maxillofacial diseases.

Author (Year)	Application	Imaging Modality	Model/Platform	Training and Validation Dataset	Test Dataset/Cross-validation	Execution Time	Performance: Deep Learning	Performance: Manual/Semi-automatic Method	Major Findings
Jaw cysts and tumors									
Lee et al. (2020) [16]	Detection, segmentation, and classification of OKCs, dentigerous and periapical cysts	Panoramic and CBCT images	CNN (Inception v3)	912 panoramic and 789 CBCT images	228 panoramic and 197 CBCT images	NA	Panoramic/CBCT AUC = 0.85/0.91 SEN = 88%/96% SPE = 77%/77%	NA	The model on CBCT images obtained higher diagnostic performance than the one on panoramic images.
Bispo et al. (2021) [17]	Differential diagnosis of ameloblastoma and OKCs	CT	CNN (Inception v3)	2500 images augmented based on 350 slices from 40 scans of patients with ameloblastoma or OKCs	2-fold CV with 5 iterations	NA	ACC = 90–92%	NA	The model obtained higher accuracy in identifying OKCs than ameloblastoma.
Chai et al. (2022) [18]	Classification of ameloblastoma and OKCs	CBCT	CNN (Inception v3)	272 scans of patients with ameloblastoma or OKCs	78 scans of patients with ameloblastoma or OKCs	Model/Senior/Junior OMF surgeons 36/1471/1113 s (78 scans)	ACC = 85% SEN = 87% SPE = 82% F1 = 85%	7 senior/30 junior OMF surgeons ACC = 66%/59% SEN = 60%/64% SPE = 71%/53% F1 = 64%/61%	The model outperformed both senior and junior OMF surgeons.
Lymph node metastasis									
Ariji et al. (2019) [22]	Differentiation of metastatic cervical lymph nodes from negative lymph nodes in OSCC patients	Contrast-enhanced CT	CNN (AlexNet)	441 cropped images including 127 metastatic and 314 non-metastatic lymph nodes from 45 OSCC patients	5-fold CV	NA	AUC = 0.80 ACC = 78% SEN = 75% SPE = 81% PPV = 80% NPV = 77%	2 radiologists AUC = 0.83 ACC = 83% SEN = 78% SPE = 89% PPV = 87% NPV = 80%	The model performed similarly to the radiologists.
Ariji et al. (2020) [23]	Differentiation between metastatic lymph nodes with and without extranodal extension in OSCC patients	Contrast-enhanced CT	CNN (AlexNet)	80% of 703 cropped images including metastatic lymph nodes with or without extranodal extension from 51 OSCC patients	20% of 703 cropped images	11 s	AUC = 0.82 ACC = 84% SEN = 67% SPE = 90% PPV = 69% NPV = 89%	4 Radiologists AUC = 0.52–63 ACC = 51–63% SEN = 42–55% SPE = 57–71% PPV = 52–66% NPV = 51–61%	The model outperformed 4 radiologists in identifying metastatic lymph nodes with extranodal extension.
Ariji et al. (2021) [24]	Detection of cervical lymph nodes in OSCC patients	Contrast-enhanced CT	CNN (DetectNet)	320 image slices including 134 metastatic and 448 non-metastatic lymph nodes from 56 OSCC patients	45 image slices including 25 metastatic and 69 non-metastatic lymph nodes from 56 OSCC patients	8 s	SEN = 73% PPV = 96% F1 = 83% False positive rates per images = 4%	NA	The model has the potential to automatically detect cervical lymph nodes.

Table 1. *Cont.*

Author (Year)	Application	Imaging Modality	Model/Platform	Training and Validation Dataset	Test Dataset/Cross-validation	Execution Time	Performance		Major Findings
							Deep Learning	Manual/Semi-automatic Method	
Ariji et al. (2022) [25]	Detection and segmentation of metastatic cervical lymph nodes in OSCC patients	Contrast-enhanced CT	CNN (U-Net)	911 image slices including 134 metastatic and 446 non-metastatic lymph nodes from 59 OSCC patients	72 image slices of 24 metastatic and 68 non-metastatic lymph nodes from 59 OSCC patients	7 s	Detection AUC = 0.95 ACC = 96% SEN = 98% SPE = 95% Segmentation SEN = 74% PPV = 94% F1 = 83%	2 radiologists Detection AUC = 0.90 ACC = 89% SEN = 94% SPE = 86%	The model outperformed 2 radiologists in detecting metastatic cervical lymph nodes while its segmentation accuracy should be improved.
Salivary gland diseases									
Kise et al. (2019) [30]	Diagnosis of Sjögren's syndrome	CT	CNN (AlexNet)	400 image slices from 20 scans of patients with Sjögren's syndrome and 20 scans of individuals without parotid gland abnormalities	100 image slices from 5 scans of patients with Sjögren's syndrome and 5 scans of individuals without parotid gland abnormalities	NA	ACC = 0.96 SEN = 100% SPE = 92%	3 experienced/3 inexperienced OMF radiologists ACC = 98%/84% SEN = 99%/78% SPE = 97%/89%	The model performed similarly to experienced radiologists and outperformed inexperienced radiologists.
Zhang et al. (2021) [32]	Classification between benign and malignant parotid gland tumors	CT	CNNs (Improved CNN, VGG16, InceptionV3, ResNet, and DenseNet)	720 image slices (group 1) and 1050 image slices (group 2)	180 image slices (group 1) and 270 image slices (group 2)	<1 min	Improved CNN on Group 1/2 ACC = 98%/78% SEN = 97%/77% SPE = 99%/79% PPV = 99%/79% F1 = 98%/78%	NA	The improved CNN model achieved the highest classification accuracy than other pre-trained CNN models.
Yuan et al. (2022) [31]	Classification between pleomorphic adenoma and malignant parotid gland tumors	CT	CNN (ResNet50)	121 scans	30 scans	NA	ACC = 90%	NA	The model achieved high accuracy in identifying malignant parotid gland tumors.
Temporomandibular disorders									
de Dumast et al. (2018) [40]	Classification of morphological variation in TMJ osteoarthritis	CBCT	Deep neural network	Scans of 259 condyles from 154/105 individuals with/without TMJ osteoarthritis	Scans of 34 condyles from 17/17 individuals with/without TMJ osteoarthritis.	NA	Agreement with two experts = 91%	NA	The model has the potential to assist clinicians in the diagnosis of TMJ osteoarthritis.

Table 1. *Cont.*

Author (Year)	Application	Imaging Modality	Model/Platform	Training and Validation Dataset	Test Dataset/Cross-validation	Execution Time	Performance: Deep Learning	Performance: Manual/Semi-automatic Method	Major Findings
Kim et al. (2021) [39]	Segmentation and measurement of the cortical thickness of mandibular condyle head	CBCT	CNN (U-Net)	11,776 image slices from 23 scans of individuals without pathological bony changes on the condyle head	1024 image slices from 2 scans of individuals without pathological bony changes on the condyle head	10–15 s	Marrow bone IoU = 0.87 HD = 0.93 mm Cortical bone IoU = 0.73 HD = 1.25 mm	NA	The model may contribute to automated quantitative analysis of the changes in bony structures of TMJ.
Le et al. (2021) [38]	Segmentation of mandibular ramus and condyle	CBCT	CNN (U-Net)	90 scans of individuals with/without osteoarthritis, obtained from multiple centers	19 scans of individuals with/without osteoarthritis, obtained from multiple centers	NA	AUC = 0.95 ACC = 100% SEN = 93% SPE = 100% F1 = 92%	NA	The model may facilitate treatment planning of TMJ degeneration.
Maxillary sinus									
Xu et al. (2020) [47]	Segmentation of the maxillary sinus	CT	CNN (V-Net)	35 scans	26 scans	<1 min	DSC = 0.94 IoU = 0.90 Precision = 94%	NA	The model achieved high segmentation accuracy.
Deng et al. (2020) [48]	Segmentation of the maxillary sinus	CT	CNN (BE-FNet)	50 scans	5-fold CV	0.5 s	DSC = 0.95 VOE = 10.2% ASD = 2.9 mm	NA	The model achieved high segmentation accuracy.
Jung et al. (2021) [49]	Segmentation of maxillary sinus lesions	CBCT	CNN (3D nnU-Net)	83 scans obtained from Korea University Anam Hospital	20 scans obtained from Korea University Anam Hospital and 20 scans from Korea University Ansan Hospital	NA	Anam Hospital DSC = 0.76 Ansan Hospital DSC = 0.54	NA	A lower segmentation accuracy of the model was found on external images.
Hung et al. (2022) [50]	Detection, segmentation, and measurement of the morphological changes of the sinus mucosa	CBCT	CNN (V-Net and SVR)	347 low-dose scans of individuals with or without morphological changes of the maxillary sinus mucosa	77 low-dose and 21 standard-dose scans of individuals with or without morphological changes of the maxillary sinus mucosa	NA	Low-dose scans AUC = 0.84–0.89 SEN = 79–81% SPE = 71–89% Standard-dose scans AUC = 0.89–0.93 SEN = 79–93% SPE = 89–93%	NA	The model performed similarly on both standard- and low-dose scans.
Fractures									
Wang et al. (2022) [53]	Detection and classification of mandibular fractures	CT	CNNs (U-Net and ResNet)	278 scans	408 scans	NA	AUC = 0.93–0.98 ACC = 94–98% SEN = 91–97% SPE = 91–99%	NA	The model may assist clinicians in timely and accurate detection of mandibular fractures.

Table 1. *Cont.*

Author (Year)	Application	Imaging Modality	Model/Platform	Training and Validation Dataset	Test Dataset/Cross-validation	Execution Time	Performance		Major Findings
							Deep Learning	Manual/Semi-automatic Method	
Dentofacial deformities and malocclusion									
Kim et al. (2020) [66]	Classification of skeletal malocclusion	CBCT	Multi-channel CNNs	173 scans of individuals with Class I, II, or III malocclusion	45 scans of individuals with Class I, II, or III malocclusion	NA	ACC = 93–94% SEN = 95% PPV = 93–94% F1 = 94–95%	NA	The model may facilitate orthodontic and orthognathic evaluation to determine whether the patient needs surgical correction.
Ma et al. (2022) [68]	Prediction of skeletal changes after orthognathic surgery	CT	CNN	50 pairs of preoperative and postoperative full skull scans	6 pairs of preoperative and postoperative full skull scans	43 s	Mean landmark localization deviation = 5.4 mm 74% of the predicted postoperative skull models was consistent with the ground truth	NA	The model may assist OMF surgeons in predicting postoperative skeletal changes for orthognathic surgical planning.
ter Horst et al. (2021) [67]	Prediction of virtual soft tissue profile after mandibular advancement surgery	3D photographs and CBCT	Autoencoder-inspired neural network	119 pairs of 3D photographs and CBCT scans of patients who underwent mandibular advancement surgery	14 pairs of 3D photographs and CBCT scans of patients who underwent mandibular advancement surgery	NA	Mean absolute error 1 mm (lower face) 1.1 mm (lower lip) 1.4 mm (chin)	MTM-based soft-tissue simulations Mean absolute error 1.5 mm (lower face) 1.7 mm (lower lip) 2 mm (chin)	The model performed similarly to the MTM-based soft-tissue simulations, indicating that it may be useful for soft tissue profile prediction in orthognathic surgery.
Lin et al. (2021) [69]	Assessment of facial symmetry before and after orthognathic surgery	CBCT	CNNs (VGG16, VGG19, ResNet50, and Xception)	71 scans	59 scans	NA	ACC 80% (VGG16) 86% (VGG19) 83% (ResNet50) 90% (Xception)	NA	The model trained with Xception achieved highest accuracy for facial symmetry assessment.
Image registration									
Chung et al. (2020) [65]	Registration between CBCT and optical dental model scans	CBCT and optical dental model scans	Deep pose regression neural networks and optimal cluster-based matching	150 pairs of CBCT and optical maxillary model scans and 150 pairs of CBCT and mandibular model scans	3-fold CV	17.6 s	Mean distance errors 5.1 mm (surface) 1.8 mm (landmarks)	Conventional three-point registration Mean distance errors 9.6 mm (surface) 2.7 mm (landmarks)	The model is applicable to full-arch scanned models and can avoid metal artifacts during the matching procedures.

Table 1. *Cont.*

Author (Year)	Application	Imaging Modality	Model/Platform	Training and Validation Dataset	Test Dataset/Cross-validation	Execution Time	Performance: Deep Learning	Performance: Manual/Semi-automatic Method	Major Findings
Jang et al. (2021) [64]	Registration between CBCT and intraoral scans	CBCT and intraoral scans	CNN	71 maxillary or mandibular intraoral scans and the corresponding 49 CBCT scans	22 pairs of CBCT and intraoral scans	NA	Mean distance errors 0.5 mm (surface) 0.2 mm (landmarks)	Manual registration Mean distance errors 1.7 mm (surface) 0.7 mm (landmarks)	The model outperformed the manual registration method.
Segmentation of maxillofacial structures									
Lo Giudice et al. (2021) [56]	Segmentation of the mandible	CBCT	CNN	20 scans	20 scans	50 s	DSC = 0.97 Matching percentage = 89%	NA	The model may be useful in the planning of maxillofacial surgical procedures.
Xu et al. (2021) [63]	Segmentation of mandibles with/without tumor invasion	CT	CNN (3D V-Net)	160 scans of 80 consisting of 80 MTI scans and 80 Non-MTI scans	70 scans consisting of 35 MTI scans and 35 Non-MTI scans	7.4 s	Non-MTI segmentation DSC = 0.98 IoU = 0.96 ASD = 0.06 mm HD = 0.48 mm MTI segmentation DSC = 0.97 IoU = 0.94 ASD = 0.16 mm HD = 1.16mm	NA	The model obtained high accuracy in segmenting mandibles with and without tumor invasion.
Sin et al. (2021) [59]	Segmentation of pharyngeal airway	CBCT	CNN (U-Net)	260 scans	46 scans	NA	DSC = 0.92 IoU = 0.99	NA	The model can efficiently calculate the pharyngeal airway volume from CBCT images.
Orhan et al. (2022) [60]	Segmentation of the pharyngeal airway in OSA and non-OSA patients	CBCT	Diagnocat (a commercially available AI platform; https://diagnocat.com (accessed on 5 December 2022))	NA	200 scans of 100 OSA and 100 non-OSA patients, taken using 3 different CBCT scanners	NA	ICC between Diagnocat and radiologists = 0.97	NA	Diagnocat performed similarly to radiologists and can efficiently calculate the pharyngeal airway volume in OSA and non-OSA patients.

Table 1. *Cont.*

Author (Year)	Application	Imaging Modality	Model/Platform	Training and Validation Dataset	Test Dataset/Cross-validation	Execution Time	Performance		Major Findings
							Deep Learning	Manual/Semi-automatic Method	
Preda et al. (2022) [57]	Segmentation of the maxillofacial complex, including palatine, maxillary, zygomatic, nasal, and lacrimal bones	CBCT	CNN (U-Net)	120 scans taken using two different scanners	24 scans taken using two different scanners	Model 39 s Manual 133 min	DSC = 0.93 IoU = 0.86 95% HD = 0.62 mm RMS 0.5 mm	Semi-automated segmentation using Mimics DSC = 0.69 IoU = 0.53 95% HD = 2.78 mm RMS 1.76 mm	The model may improve the efficiency of the digital workflows for patient-specific treatment planning of maxillofacial surgical procedures.
Ezhov et al. (2021) [58]	Segmentation of teeth and jaws, numbering of teeth, detection of caries, periapical lesions, and periodontitis	CBCT	Diagnocat (a commercially available AI platform; https://diagnocat.com (accessed on 5 December 2022))	1346 scans taken using 17 scanners	30 scans	With the aid of Diagnocat = 17.6 min Without the aid of Diagnocat = 18.7 min	Diagnocat SEN = 92% SPE = 99% 12 dentists with the aid of Diagnocat SEN = 85% SPE = 97%	4 OMF radiologists SEN = 93–94% SPE = 99–100% 12 dentists without the aid of Diagnocat SEN = 77% SPE = 96%	Diagnocat performed similarly to four radiologists and improved twelve dentists' performance
Jaskari et al. (2020) [61]	Segmentation of the mandibular canal	CBCT	CNN	509 scans taken using two scanners	15 scans	NA	MCD = 0.56 mm ASSD = 0.45 mm DSC = 0.57 (left) and 0.58 (right) HD = 1.40 (left) and 1.38 (right)	NA	The model may help to locate the inferior alveolar nerve for surgical planning
Lim et al. (2021) [62]	Segmentation of the mandibular canal	CBCT	CNN (3D nnU-Net)	83 scans from Korea University Anam Hospital	15, 20, and 20 scans from Korea University Anam Hospital (1), Korea University Ansan Hospital (2), and Korea University Guro Hospital (3)	Model 86 s Manual 125 s	Internal testing DSC = 0.58 (1) External testing DSC = 0.55 (2) DSC = 0.43 (3)	NA	The model may help to locate the inferior alveolar nerve for surgical planning

Abbreviations: 3D, three-dimensional; ACC, accuracy; ASSD, average symmetric surface distance; AUC, area under the ROC curve; CBCT/CT, cone-beam computed tomography; CMS, contour matching score; CNN, convolutional neural network; CV, cross-validation; DSC, dice similarity coefficient; F1, F1-score; HD, hausdorff distance; IoU, intersection over union; JSC, jaccard similarity coefficient; k-NN, k-nearest neighbors; OKC, odontogenic keratocyst; LDA, linear discriminant analysis; LOOCV, leave-one-out cross-validation; MCD, mean curve distance; MTM, mass tensor model; MTI, mandible with tumor invasion; NA, not available; NN, neural network; NPV, negative predictive value; OMF, oral and maxillofacial; OSA, obstructive sleep apnea; OSCC, oral squamous cell carcinoma; PPV, positive predictive value (precision); RMS, root mean square; SDA, sparse discriminant analysis; SEN, sensitivity (recall); SPE, specificity; SSIM, structural similarity index measure; SVM, support vector machine; TMJ, temporomandibular joint; VOE, volumetric overlap error.

Table 2. Performance of radiomics models on CT/CBCT images for maxillofacial diseases.

Author (Year)	Application	Imaging Modality	Image Dataset	Region of Interest for Feature Extraction	Data for Model Building	Machine Learning Approach	Validation Method	Performance of the Best Model(s)	Major Findings
Zhong et al. (2021) [27]	Prediction of cervical lymph node metastasis in patients with tongue cancer	Contrast-enhanced CT	313 scans of patients with tongue cancer	Primary cancer	Radiomic features and clinical lymph node status	Artificial neural network	Hold-out validation (20%)	Model on radiomic features and clinical lymph node status AUC = 0.94 ACC = 84% SEN = 93% SPE = 77% Model on radiomic features AUC = 0.92 ACC = 86% SEN = 82% SPE = 89%	The model on radiomic features and clinical lymph node status achieved higher prediction accuracy than the one only on radiomic features.
Kubo et al. (2022) [26]	Prediction of occult cervical lymph node metastasis in patients with tongue cancer	Contrast-enhanced CT	161 scans of tongue cancer patients with or without occult cervical lymph node metastasis	Cervical lymph nodes	Radiomic features	kNN, SVM, CART, RF, AdaBoost with/without SMOTE	10-fold CV	Side level RF with SMOTE AUC = 0.92 ACC = 85% SEN = 82% PPV = 88% Region level SVM with SMOTE AUC = 0.98 ACC = 96% SEN = 95% PPV = 96%	The radiomics models may serve as useful tools to support clinical decision making in the management of patients with tongue cancer.
Morgan et al. (2021) [28]	Prediction of local failure in head and neck cancer	Contrast-enhanced CT and CBCT	Baseline CT scan, two CBCT scans at fractions 1 and 21 of radiotherapy from 90 head and neck SCC patients with or without local failure	All primary and nodal structures	Radiomic features and several clinical variables	Explainable boosting machine with 25 iterations	5-fold CV	Fused ensemble model (primary/nodal structures) AUC = 0.87/0.91 SEN = 78%/100% SPE = 91%/68%	The model on radiomic features and clinical variables achieved the highest accuracy in predicting local failure in head and neck cancer.

Table 2. *Cont.*

Author (Year)	Application	Imaging Modality	Image Dataset	Region of Interest for Feature Extraction	Data for Model Building	Machine Learning Approach	Validation Method	Performance of the Best Model(s)	Major Findings
Xu et al. (2021) [34]	Differentiation between benign and malignant parotid gland tumors	CT	87 scans of patients with benign or malignant parotid gland tumor	Primary tumors	Radiomic features and radiological variables including the location and metastases of lymph nodes	SVM	Hold-out validation (38 scans)	The combined model AUC = 0.84 SEN = 82% SPE = 74% The model on radiomic features AUC = 0.77 SEN = 79% SPE = 89%	The combined model outperformed the models on individual radiomic features, lymph node location, or lymph node metastases.
Zhang et al. (2021) [33]	Differentiation between low- and high-grade mucoepider-moid carcinoma of the salivary glands	CT	53 scans of patients with low or high grade mucoepidermoid carcinoma	Primary cancer	Radiomic features	Logistic regression	NA	AUC = 0.80 ACC = 78% SEN = 89% PPV = 67%	High-grade mucoepidermoid carcinomas may be associated with a low energy, high correlation texture, and high surface irregularity.
Liu et al. (2021) [35]	Differentiation between pleomorphic adenoma and Warthin tumors of the parotid glands	CT and MRI	659 pairs of CT and MRI scans from patients with pleomorphic adenoma or Warthin tumors	Primary tumors	CT- and MRI-derived radiomic features	Logistic regression	NA	CT/MRI AUC = 0.88/0.91 ACC = 78%/84% SEN = 81%/85% SPE = 76%/83% PPV = 70%/77% NPV = 86%/89%	The model on MRI-derived radiomic features performed slightly higher than but not significantly differently from the model on CT-derived radiomic features.
Bianchi et al. (2020) [41]	Diagnosis of TMJ osteoarthritis	CBCT	92 scans of subjects with or without TMJ osteoarthritis	Internal condylar lateral region	20 radiomic and 25 biomolecular features, 5 clinical and 2 demographic variables	LR, RF, LightGBM, XGBoost with 10 iterations	5-fold CV	XGBoost + LightGBM AUC = 0.87 ACC = 82% SEN = 84% F1 = 82%	The model may be helpful for screening individuals with early TMJ osteoarthritis.

Abbreviations: ACC, accuracy; AUC, area under the ROC curve; CART, classification and regression tree; CBCT/CT, cone-beam computed tomography; CV, cross-validation; F1, F1-score; LASSO, least absolute shrinkage and selection operator; LightGBM, light gradient boosting machine; LR, logistic regression; mRMR, maximum relevance and minimum redundancy; kNN, k-nearest neighbor; ICC, intra-class correlation coefficient; MRI, magnetic resonance imaging; PPV, positive predictive value (precision); RF, random forest; RFE, recursive feature elimination; SCC, squamous cell carcinoma; SEN, sensitivity (recall); SMOTE, synthetic minority oversampling technique; SPE, specificity; SVM, support vector machine; TMJ, temporomandibular joint; U test, Mann–Whitney U test; XGBoost, extreme gradient boosting.

3. The Challenges and Prospects of Deep Learning and Radiomics on CT/CBCT for Maxillofacial Diseases

Based on current evidence, early diagnosis, accurate prognostic prediction, and efficient treatment planning are main focuses of deep learning and radiomics models developed on CT/CBCT for maxillofacial diseases (Tables 1 and 2). Few studies reported that deep learning models on CBCT images performed better than those on 2D radiographic images [3,16]. These findings may result from more informative features on CBCT than on 2D images to be utilized for training the models. Most of the proposed deep learning models showed high performance, and some of them even outperformed human experts, especially when the ground truth was not based solely on visual inspection on radiographic images. Deep learning models capable of detecting diseases, particularly malignant lesions, at an early stage are expected to allow for the earliest possible diagnosis and treatment to prevent disease progression, which therefore will improve treatment outcome and prognosis. Apart from diagnostic applications, deep learning models were also developed to assist clinicians in many time-consuming tasks required in the treatment planning process for patients with maxillofacial diseases as mentioned above. Applications for automated multimodal image registration as well as localization, segmentation, and measurement of anatomical structures or pathologies on CT/CBCT images have the potential to improve the accuracy and efficiency of digital workflows for patient-specific treatment planning, which may enable a more precise and personalized approach for the management of maxillofacial diseases.

Despite the promising performance of deep learning models proposed, their generalizability has not been validated sufficiently. Most of them were trained using CT/CBCT images acquired at a certain time point from a single institution and were tested with the cross-validation or split sample validation method using images from the same institution, which is very likely to cause overfitting of the trained model. Some studies have reported that their models had inferior performance when tested on images from other institutions [70,71]. More validation studies that prospectively collect new datasets to test the performance of the developed models are needed. Ideally, the model's performance should be evaluated on external image data, acquired with different scanners and imaging protocols, from multiple institutions to verify their true generalizability. If the model's performance on external datasets is not favorable, the datasets from different centers should be included for cross-center training to avoid overfitting and improve the model's generalizability. On the other hand, training data insufficiency is also one of the most common reasons that cause overfitting, resulting in the model's learning statistical regularity specific to the training data. Some strategical learning approaches, such as federated learning and learning from the normal methods, may be the solution to overcome the insufficiency of training data [72]. Moreover, it has been raised that radiomic analysis is more robust than deep learning approach in the case of training with small data [73]. Incorporating radiomic features into deep learning models seems to be able to avoid overfitting [73].

Deep learning algorithms allow for automatic extraction and selection of imaging features on radiographic images in the neural network. As deep learning models automatically extract hierarchical features in complex data and optimize the weighted parameters from raw data, their decision-making process cannot be deduced, and thus, they are considered as "black-box" models (Figure 3). Compared with deep learning models, radiomics models have been seen as "glass-box" models because of better transparency [28]. The radiomics approach involves the extraction of quantitative imaging features from the segmented regions of interest on radiographic images, selection of reproducible and reliable features, and building a high-level statistical model with the selected features using machine learning methods for diagnostic and predictive purposes. Therefore, the contribution of each selected feature to the overall prediction can be deduced from radiomics models, which is one of the main advantages of radiomic analysis as compared to deep learning [28]. Thus far, radiomics studies on CT/CBCT were conducted mainly for differentiating between benign and malignant lesions as well as predicting cervical lymph node metastasis and local failure in patients with oral, head and neck cancer. There are still several challenges in current radiomics studies regarding the repeatability and reproducibility of radiomic features and the stability of feature selection [74–76]. The variations in the scanners, imaging protocols, and reconstruction algorithms may affect the repeatability and reproducibility of radiomic features [77]. Moreover, radiomics models built based on an unstable feature selection method may include many unstable features, resulting in a lack of reliability of the developed models and reduced accuracy on external data. The use of ensemble methods, including resampling, bagging, and boosting techniques, for radiomic feature selection has been highly recommended to improve the stability of radiomic feature selection [28,78]. Regardless, radiomic models also have some limitations when compared to deep learning methods, such as the requirement of segmentation, and its application is limited to classification of segmented lesions. These limitations may be overcome by integrating radiomics and deep learning to expand their clinical applications.

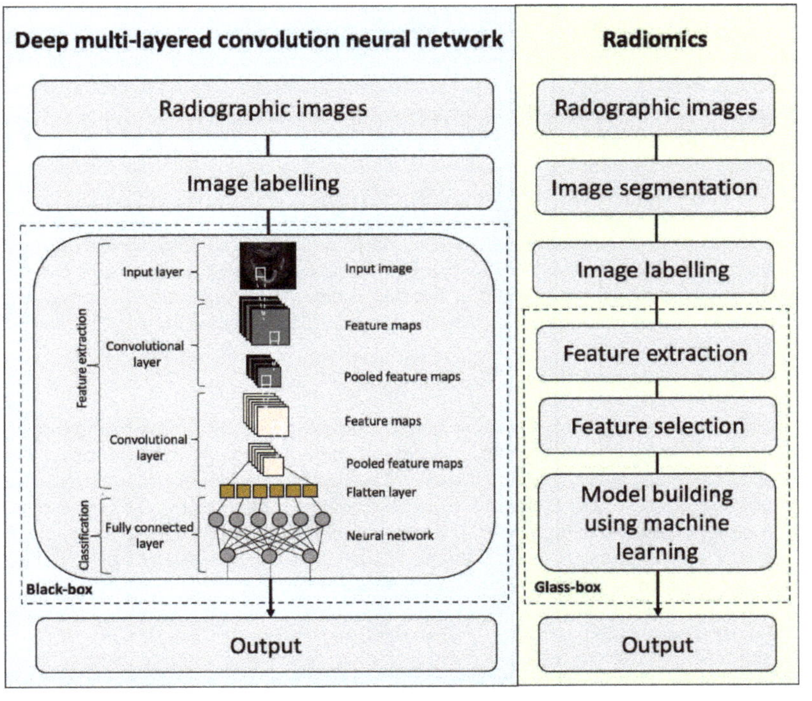

Figure 3. Flowchart demonstrating the main differences in the workflow between deep learning and radiomics in radiological studies.

It remains unknown whether CT- and CBCT-derived radiomic features are interchangeable. Few studies have assessed the differences in radiomic feature values of head and neck cancer between CT and CBCT images of the same individuals [79,80]. It was reported that no significant differences were found in most of the extracted feature values between the paired CT and CBCT images, indicating that radiomic features from CT and CBCT may be interchangeable [79]. Notably, some image processing techniques, such as high-pass filtering, could affect the reproducibility of radiomic features [79]. On the contrary, some held the view that radiomic features from CBCT may not be directly transferable to those from CT due to the differences in their inherent image characteristics, such as the scatters, noise, and resolution [80]. These differences may contribute to larger variations in radiomic feature values calculated from specific regions of interest between the two imaging modalities. The analysis of delta radiomic features (i.e., the changes in radiomic feature values from serial scans) may be the solution to improve the reproducibility of radiomic features for the management of oral, head and neck cancer [80].

The reproducibility in the radiomic feature values calculated by different software packages (such as Pyradiomics, MaZda, LIFEx, MITK Phenotyping, and CERR radiomic extension) remains uncertain. Some found that the values of features in certain categories (e.g., second-order features) were not consistent across packages [81] while others reported high consistency [82]. Researchers should be aware of this issue when comparing results from studies using different radiomics software packages. The image biomarker standardization initiative (IBSI; https://ibsi.readthedocs.io/ (accessed on 5 December 2022)) is an independent international collaboration where experts in various areas of medical imaging from several institutions in eight countries work together to standardize the extraction of image biomarkers (i.e., radiomic features) from diagnostic imaging for the purpose of achieving greater harmonization of radiomics research [83]. Standardization of radiomic analysis is fundamental for the comparison and validation of findings from different studies and is crucial for a possible translation of radiomics into clinical practice.

At present, most of the deep learning and radiomics models for maxillofacial diseases were developed based solely on CT/CBCT image data. Enriching these models with diverse data from the individual level (such as demographic, behavioral, and social characteristics), setting level (such as geospatial, environmental, or provider-related data), and system level (such as health insurance, regulatory, and legislative data) may facilitate a deeper and more holistic understanding of individual health and disease and may therefore enable a more precise and personalized management of patients with maxillofacial diseases [84]. Most importantly, the true usefulness and cost-effectiveness of these deep learning and radiomics models in daily practice should be further assessed to gain the trust of patients, providers, and healthcare organizers. Further development of explainable AI systems that can provide an insight of how the predictions are made is the key to fostering trust in their clinical use [73].

4. Conclusions

A wide range of deep learning and radiomic models on CT/CBCT have been proposed for automatic diagnosis, segmentation, and classification of jaw cysts and tumors, cervical lymph node metastasis, salivary gland diseases, TMJ disorders, maxillary sinus pathologies, mandibular fractures, and dentomaxillofacial deformities. The models with performance on par with specialists have the potential to serve as clinically practicable tools to achieve the earliest possible diagnosis and treatment, leading to a more precise and personalized approach for the management of maxillofacial diseases.

Author Contributions: K.F.H., writing—original draft preparation; Q.Y.H.A., L.M.W., A.W.K.Y., D.T.S.L. and Y.Y.L., writing—review and editing. All authors have read and agreed to the published version of the manuscript.

Funding: This research received no external funding.

Conflicts of Interest: The authors declare no conflict of interest.

References

1. Joda, T.; Yeung, A.W.K.; Hung, K.; Zitzmann, N.U.; Bornstein, M.M. Disruptive innovation in dentistry: What it is and what could be next. *J. Dent. Res.* **2021**, *100*, 448–453. [CrossRef]
2. Schwendicke, F.; Samek, W.; Krois, J. Artificial intelligence in dentistry: Chances and challenges. *J. Dent. Res.* **2020**, *99*, 769–774. [CrossRef]
3. Hung, K.F.; Ai, Q.Y.H.; Leung, Y.Y.; Yeung, A.W.K. Potential and impact of artificial intelligence algorithms in dento-maxillofacial radiology. *Clin. Oral Investig.* **2022**, *26*, 5535–5555. [CrossRef]
4. Stone, P.; Brooks, R.; Brynjolfsson, E.; Calo, R.; Etzioni, O.; Hager, G.; Hirschberg, J.; Kalyanakrishnan, S.; Kamar, E.; Kraus, S.; et al. *Artificial Intelligence and Life in 2030. One Hundred Year Study on Artificial Intelligence: Report of the 2015–2016 Study Panel;* Stanford University: Stanford, CA, USA, 2016; Available online: http://ai100stanfordedu/2016-report (accessed on 5 December 2022).
5. Leite, A.F.; Vasconcelos, K.F.; Willems, H.; Jacobs, R. Radiomics and machine learning in oral healthcare. *Proteom. Clin. Appl.* **2020**, *14*, e1900040. [CrossRef]

6. van Timmeren, J.E.; Cester, D.; Tanadini-Lang, S.; Alkadhi, H.; Baessler, B. Radiomics in medical imaging-"how-to" guide and critical reflection. *Insights Imaging* **2020**, *11*, 91. [CrossRef]
7. Roy, S.; Whitehead, T.D.; Quirk, J.D.; Salter, A.; Ademuyiwa, F.O.; Li, S.; An, H.; Shoghi, K.I. Optimal co-clinical radiomics: Sensitivity of radiomic features to tumour volume, image noise and resolution in co-clinical T1-weighted and T2-weighted magnetic resonance imaging. *EBioMedicine* **2020**, *59*, 102963. [CrossRef]
8. Roy, S.; Whitehead, T.D.; Li, S.; Ademuyiwa, F.O.; Wahl, R.L.; Dehdashti, F.; Shoghi, K.I. Co-clinical FDG-PET radiomic signature in predicting response to neoadjuvant chemotherapy in triple-negative breast cancer. *Eur. J. Nucl. Med. Mol. Imaging* **2021**, *49*, 550–562. [CrossRef]
9. Hung, K.; Yeung, A.W.K.; Tanaka, R.; Bornstein, M.M. Current applications, opportunities, and limitations of AI for 3D imaging in dental research and practice. *Int. J. Environ. Res. Public Health* **2020**, *17*, 4424. [CrossRef] [PubMed]
10. Hung, K.; Montalvao, C.; Tanaka, R.; Kawai, T.; Bornstein, M.M. The use and performance of artificial intelligence applications in dental and maxillofacial radiology: A systematic review. *Dentomaxillofac. Radiol.* **2020**, *49*, 20190107. [CrossRef]
11. Poedjiastoeti, W.; Suebnukarn, S. Application of convolutional neural network in the diagnosis of jaw tumors. *Healthc. Inform. Res.* **2018**, *24*, 236–241. [CrossRef]
12. Kwon, O.; Yong, T.H.; Kang, S.R.; Kim, J.E.; Huh, K.H.; Heo, M.S. Automatic diagnosis for cysts and tumors of both jaws on panoramic radiographs using a deep convolution neural network. *Dentomaxillofac. Radiol.* **2020**, *49*, 20200185. [CrossRef]
13. Endres, M.G.; Hillen, F.; Salloumis, M.; Sedaghat, A.R.; Niehues, S.M.; Quatela, O.; Hanken, H.; Smeets, R.; Beck-Broichsitter, B.; Rendenbach, C.; et al. Development of a deep learning algorithm for periapical disease detection in dental radiographs. *Diagnostics* **2020**, *10*, 430. [CrossRef]
14. Ariji, Y.; Yanashita, Y.; Kutsuna, S.; Muramatsu, C.; Fukuda, M.; Kise, Y.; Nozawa, M.; Kuwada, C.; Fujita, H.; Katsumata, A.; et al. Automatic detection and classification of radiolucent lesions in the mandible on panoramic radiographs using a deep learning object detection technique. *Oral Surg. Oral Med. Oral Pathol. Oral Radiol.* **2019**, *128*, 424–430. [CrossRef]
15. Watanabe, H.; Ariji, Y.; Fukuda, M.; Kuwada, C.; Kise, Y.; Nozawa, M.; Sugita, Y.; Ariji, E. Deep learning object detection of maxillary cyst-like lesions on panoramic radiographs: Preliminary study. *Oral Radiol.* **2021**, *37*, 487–493. [CrossRef] [PubMed]
16. Lee, J.H.; Kim, D.H.; Jeong, S.N. Diagnosis of cystic lesions using panoramic and cone beam computed tomographic images based on deep learning neural network. *Oral Dis.* **2020**, *26*, 152–158. [CrossRef]
17. Bispo, M.S.; Pierre Júnior, M.L.G.Q.; Apolinário Jr, A.L.; Dos Santos, J.N.; Junior, B.C.; Neves, F.S.; Crusoé-Rebello, I. Computer tomographic differential diagnosis of ameloblastoma and odontogenic keratocyst: Classification using a convolutional neural network. *Dentomaxillofac. Radiol.* **2021**, *50*, 20210002. [CrossRef] [PubMed]
18. Chai, Z.K.; Mao, L.; Chen, H.; Sun, T.G.; Shen, X.M.; Liu, J.; Sun, Z.J. Improved diagnostic accuracy of ameloblastoma and odontogenic keratocyst on cone-beam CT by artificial intelligence. *Front Oncol.* **2022**, *11*, 793417. [CrossRef] [PubMed]
19. Negi, A.; Puri, A.; Gupta, R.; Nangia, R.; Sachdeva, A.; Mittal, M. Comparison of immunohistochemical expression of antiapoptotic protein survivin in normal oral mucosa, oral leukoplakia, and oral squamous cell carcinoma. *Patholog. Res. Int.* **2015**, *2015*, 840739. [CrossRef] [PubMed]
20. Hanai, N.; Asakage, T.; Kiyota, N.; Homma, A.; Hayashi, R. Controversies in relation to neck management in N0 early oral tongue cancer. *Jpn. J. Clin. Oncol.* **2019**, *49*, 297–305. [CrossRef]
21. van den Brekel, M.W.; Stel, H.V.; Castelijns, J.A.; Nauta, J.J.; van der Waal, I.; Valk, J.; Meyer, C.J.; Snow, G.B. Cervical lymph node metastasis: Assessment of radiologic criteria. *Radiology* **1990**, *177*, 379–384. [CrossRef]
22. Ariji, Y.; Fukuda, M.; Kise, Y.; Nozawa, M.; Yanashita, Y.; Fujita, H.; Katsumata, A.; Ariji, E. Contrast-enhanced computed tomography image assessment of cervical lymph node metastasis in patients with oral cancer by using a deep learning system of artificial intelligence. *Oral Surg. Oral Med. Oral Pathol. Oral Radiol.* **2019**, *127*, 458–463. [CrossRef] [PubMed]
23. Ariji, Y.; Sugita, Y.; Nagao, T.; Nakayama, A.; Fukuda, M.; Kise, Y.; Nozawa, M.; Nishiyama, M.; Katumata, A.; Ariji, E. CT evaluation of extranodal extension of cervical lymph node metastases in patients with oral squamous cell carcinoma using deep learning classification. *Oral Radiol.* **2020**, *36*, 148–155. [CrossRef] [PubMed]
24. Ariji, Y.; Fukuda, M.; Nozawa, M.; Kuwada, C.; Goto, M.; Ishibashi, K.; Nakayama, A.; Sugita, Y.; Nagao, T.; Ariji, E. Automatic detection of cervical lymph nodes in patients with oral squamous cell carcinoma using a deep learning technique: A preliminary study. *Oral Radiol.* **2021**, *37*, 290–296. [CrossRef] [PubMed]
25. Ariji, Y.; Kise, Y.; Fukuda, M.; Kuwada, C.; Ariji, E. Segmentation of metastatic cervical lymph nodes from CT images of oral cancers using deep-learning technology. *Dentomaxillofac. Radiol.* **2022**, *51*, 20210515. [CrossRef]
26. Kubo, K.; Kawahara, D.; Murakami, Y.; Takeuchi, Y.; Katsuta, T.; Imano, N.; Nishibuchi, I.; Saito, A.; Konishi, M.; Kakimoto, N.; et al. Development of a radiomics and machine learning model for predicting occult cervical lymph node metastasis in patients with tongue cancer. *Oral Surg. Oral Med. Oral Pathol. Oral Radiol.* **2022**, *134*, 93–101. [CrossRef]
27. Zhong, Y.W.; Jiang, Y.; Dong, S.; Wu, W.J.; Wang, L.X.; Zhang, J.; Huang, M.W. Tumor radiomics signature for artificial neural network-assisted detection of neck metastasis in patient with tongue cancer. *J. Neuroradiol.* **2022**, *49*, 213–218. [CrossRef]
28. Morgan, H.E.; Wang, K.; Dohopolski, M.; Liang, X.; Folkert, M.R.; Sher, D.J.; Wang, J. Exploratory ensemble interpretable model for predicting local failure in head and neck cancer: The additive benefit of CT and intra-treatment cone-beam computed tomography features. *Quant. Imaging Med. Surg.* **2021**, *11*, 4781–4796. [CrossRef]
29. Gündüz, E.; Alçin, Ö.F.; Kizilay, A.; Piazza, C. Radiomics and deep learning approach to the differential diagnosis of parotid gland tumors. *Curr. Opin. Otolaryngol. Head Neck Surg.* **2022**, *30*, 107–113. [CrossRef]

30. Kise, Y.; Ikeda, H.; Fujii, T.; Fukuda, M.; Ariji, Y.; Fujita, H.; Katsumata, A.; Ariji, E. Preliminary study on the application of deep learning system to diagnosis of Sjögren's syndrome on CT images. *Dentomaxillofac. Radiol.* **2019**, *48*, 20190019. [CrossRef]
31. Yuan, J.; Fan, Y.; Lv, X.; Chen, C.; Li, D.; Hong, Y.; Wang, Y. Research on the practical classification and privacy protection of CT images of parotid tumors based on ResNet50 model. *J. Phys. Conf. Ser. 2020* **2022**, *1576*, 012040. [CrossRef]
32. Zhang, H.; Lai, H.; Wang, Y.; Lv, X.; Hong, Y.; Peng, J.; Zhang, Z.; Chen, C.; Chen, C. Research on the classification of benign and malignant parotid tumors based on transfer learning and a convolutional neural network. *IEEE Access* **2021**, *9*, 40360–40371. [CrossRef]
33. Zhang, M.H.; Hasse, A.; Carroll, T.; Pearson, A.T.; Cipriani, N.A.; Ginat, D.T. Differentiating low and high grade mucoepidermoid carcinoma of the salivary glands using CT radiomics. *Gland Surg.* **2021**, *10*, 1646–1654. [CrossRef] [PubMed]
34. Xu, Y.; Shu, Z.; Song, G.; Liu, Y.; Pang, P.; Wen, X.; Gong, X. The role of preoperative computed tomography radiomics in distinguishing benign and malignant tumors of the parotid gland. *Front. Oncol.* **2021**, *11*, 634452. [CrossRef] [PubMed]
35. Liu, Y.; Zheng, J.; Lu, X.; Wang, Y.; Meng, F.; Zhao, J.; Guo, C.; Yu, L.; Zhu, Z.; Zhang, T. Radiomics-based comparison of MRI and CT for differentiating pleomorphic adenomas and Warthin tumors of the parotid gland: A retrospective study. *Oral Surg. Oral Med. Oral Pathol. Oral Radiol.* **2021**, *131*, 591–599. [CrossRef]
36. Li, D.T.S.; Leung, Y.Y. Temporomandibular disorders: Current concepts and controversies in diagnosis and management. *Diagnostics* **2021**, *11*, 459. [CrossRef]
37. Ottersen, M.K.; Abrahamsson, A.K.; Larheim, T.A.; Arvidsson, L.Z. CBCT characteristics and interpretation challenges of temporomandibular joint osteoarthritis in a hand osteoarthritis cohort. *Dentomaxillofac. Radiol.* **2019**, *48*, 20180245. [CrossRef]
38. Le, C.; Deleat-Besson, R.; Prieto, J.; Brosset, S.; Dumont, M.; Zhang, W.; Cevidanes, L.; Bianchi, J.; Ruellas, A.; Gomes, L.; et al. Automatic segmentation of mandibular ramus and condyles. In Proceedings of the 2021 43rd Annual International Conference of the IEEE Engineering in Medicine & Biology Society (EMBC), Guadalajara, Mexico, 1–5 November 2021; pp. 2952–2955.
39. Kim, Y.H.; Shin, J.Y.; Lee, A.; Park, S.; Han, S.S.; Hwang, H.J. Automated cortical thickness measurement of the mandibular condyle head on CBCT images using a deep learning method. *Sci. Rep.* **2021**, *11*, 14852. [CrossRef]
40. de Dumast, P.; Mirabel, C.; Cevidanes, L.; Ruellas, A.; Yatabe, M.; Ioshida, M.; Ribera, N.T.; Michoud, L.; Gomes, L.; Huang, C.; et al. A web-based system for neural network based classification in temporomandibular joint osteoarthritis. *Comput. Med. Imaging Graph.* **2018**, *67*, 45–54. [CrossRef]
41. Bianchi, J.; de Oliveira Ruellas, A.C.; Gonçalves, J.R.; Paniagua, B.; Prieto, J.C.; Styner, M.; Li, T.; Zhu, H.; Sugai, J.; Giannobile, W.; et al. Osteoarthritis of the Temporomandibular Joint can be diagnosed earlier using biomarkers and machine learning. *Sci. Rep.* **2020**, *10*, 8012. [CrossRef]
42. Hung, K.F.; Hui, L.L.; Leung, Y.Y. Patient-specific estimation of the bone graft volume needed for maxillary sinus floor elevation: A radiographic study using cone-beam computed tomography. *Clin. Oral Investig.* **2022**, *26*, 3875–3884. [CrossRef]
43. Yeung, A.W.K.; Hung, K.F.; Li, D.T.S.; Leung, Y.Y. The use of CBCT in evaluating the health and pathology of the maxillary sinus. *Diagnostics* **2022**, *12*, 2819. [CrossRef]
44. Hung, K.; Hui, L.; Yeung, A.W.K.; Wu, Y.; Hsung, R.T.; Bornstein, M.M. Volumetric analysis of mucous retention cysts in the maxillary sinus: A retrospective study using cone-beam computed tomography. *Imaging Sci. Dent.* **2021**, *51*, 117–127. [CrossRef]
45. Hung, K.; Montalvao, C.; Yeung, A.W.K.; Li, G.; Bornstein, M.M. Frequency, location, and morphology of accessory maxillary sinus ostia: A retrospective study using cone beam computed tomography (CBCT). *Surg. Radiol. Anat.* **2020**, *42*, 219–228. [CrossRef]
46. Yeung, A.W.K.; Colsoul, N.; Montalvao, C.; Hung, K.; Jacobs, R.; Bornstein, M.M. Visibility, location, and morphology of the primary maxillary sinus ostium and presence of accessory ostia: A retrospective analysis using cone beam computed tomography (CBCT). *Clin. Oral Investig.* **2019**, *23*, 3977–3986. [CrossRef]
47. Xu, J.; Wang, S.; Zhou, Z.; Liu, J.; Jiang, X.; Chen, X. Automatic CT image segmentation of maxillary sinus based on VGG network and improved V-Net. *Int. J. Comput. Assist. Radiol. Surg.* **2020**, *15*, 1457–1465. [CrossRef]
48. Deng, Z.; Wang, B.; Zhu, Z. BE-FNet: 3D bounding box estimation feature pyramid network for accurate and efficient maxillary sinus segmentation. *Math. Probl. Eng.* **2020**, *2020*, 5689301. [CrossRef]
49. Jung, S.K.; Lim, H.K.; Lee, S.; Cho, Y.; Song, I.S. Deep active learning for automatic segmentation of maxillary sinus lesions using a convolutional neural network. *Diagnostics* **2021**, *11*, 688. [CrossRef]
50. Hung, K.F.; Ai, Q.Y.H.; King, A.D.; Bornstein, M.M.; Wong, L.M.; Leung, Y.Y. Automatic detection and segmentation of morphological changes of the maxillary sinus mucosa on cone-beam computed tomography images using a three-dimensional convolutional neural network. *Clin. Oral Investig.* **2022**, *26*, 3987–3998. [CrossRef]
51. Hung, K.F.; Hui, L.; Yeung, A.W.K.; Jacobs, R.; Leung, Y.Y.; Bornstein, M.M. An analysis of patient dose received during cone-beam computed tomography in relation to scan settings and imaging indications as seen in a dental institution in order to establish institutional diagnostic reference levels. *Dentomaxillofac. Radiol.* **2022**, *51*, 20200529. [CrossRef]
52. Bornstein, M.M.; Yeung, A.W.K.; Tanaka, R.; von Arx, T.; Jacobs, R.; Khong, P.L. Evaluation of health or pathology of bilateral maxillary sinuses in patients referred for cone beam computed tomography using a low-dose protocol. *Int. J. Periodontics Restor. Dent.* **2018**, *38*, 699–710. [CrossRef]
53. Wang, X.; Xu, Z.; Tong, Y.; Xia, L.; Jie, B.; Ding, P.; Bai, H.; Zhang, Y.; He, Y. Detection and classification of mandibular fracture on CT scan using deep convolutional neural network. *Clin. Oral Investig.* **2022**, *26*, 4593–4601. [CrossRef]

54. Apostolakis, D.; Michelinakis, G.; Kamposiora, P.; Papavasiliou, G. The current state of computer assisted orthognathic surgery: A narrative review. *J. Dent.* **2022**, *119*, 104052. [CrossRef]
55. Shujaat, S.; Bornstein, M.M.; Price, J.B.; Jacobs, R. Integration of imaging modalities in digital dental workflows—Possibilities, limitations, and potential future developments. *Dentomaxillofac. Radiol.* **2021**, *50*, 20210268. [CrossRef]
56. Lo Giudice, A.; Ronsivalle, V.; Spampinato, C.; Leonardi, R. Fully automatic segmentation of the mandible based on convolutional neural networks (CNNs). *Orthod. Craniofac. Res.* **2021**, *24* (Suppl. S2), 100–107. [CrossRef]
57. Preda, F.; Morgan, N.; Van Gerven, A.; Nogueira-Reis, F.; Smolders, A.; Wang, X.; Nomidis, S.; Shaheen, E.; Willems, H.; Jacobs, R. Deep convolutional neural network-based automated segmentation of the maxillofacial complex from cone-beam computed tomography: A validation study. *J. Dent.* **2022**, *124*, 104238. [CrossRef]
58. Ezhov, M.; Gusarev, M.; Golitsyna, M.; Yates, J.M.; Kushnerev, E.; Tamimi, D.; Aksoy, S.; Shumilov, E.; Sanders, A.; Orhan, K. Clinically applicable artificial intelligence system for dental diagnosis with CBCT. *Sci. Rep.* **2021**, *11*, 15006. [CrossRef]
59. Sin, Ç.; Akkaya, N.; Aksoy, S.; Orhan, K.; Öz, U. A deep learning algorithm proposal to automatic pharyngeal airway detection and segmentation on CBCT images. *Orthod. Craniofac. Res.* **2021**, *24* (Suppl. S2), 117–123. [CrossRef]
60. Orhan, K.; Shamshiev, M.; Ezhov, M.; Plaksin, A.; Kurbanova, A.; Ünsal, G.; Gusarev, M.; Golitsyna, M.; Aksoy, S.; Mısırlı, M.; et al. AI-based automatic segmentation of craniomaxillofacial anatomy from CBCT scans for automatic detection of pharyngeal airway evaluations in OSA patients. *Sci. Rep.* **2022**, *12*, 11863. [CrossRef]
61. Jaskari, J.; Sahlsten, J.; Järnstedt, J.; Mehtonen, H.; Karhu, K.; Sundqvist, O.; Hietanen, A.; Varjonen, V.; Mattila, V.; Kaski, K. Deep learning method for mandibular canal segmentation in dental cone beam computed tomography volumes. *Sci. Rep.* **2020**, *10*, 5842. [CrossRef]
62. Lim, H.K.; Jung, S.K.; Kim, S.H.; Cho, Y.; Song, I.S. Deep semi-supervised learning for automatic segmentation of inferior alveolar nerve using a convolutional neural network. *BMC Oral Health* **2021**, *21*, 630. [CrossRef]
63. Xu, J.; Liu, J.; Zhang, D.; Zhou, Z.; Zhang, C.; Chen, X. A 3D segmentation network of mandible from CT scan with combination of multiple convolutional modules and edge supervision in mandibular reconstruction. *Comput. Biol. Med.* **2021**, *138*, 104925. [CrossRef]
64. Jang, T.J.; Yun, H.S.; Kim, J.E.; Lee, S.H.; Seo, J.K. Fully automatic integration of dental CBCT images and full-arch intraoral impressions with stitching error correction via individual tooth segmentation and identification. *arXiv* **2021**, arXiv:2112.01784.
65. Chung, M.; Lee, J.; Song, W.; Song, Y.; Yang, L.-H.; Lee, J.; Shin, Y.-G. Automatic registration between dental cone-beam CT and scanned surface via deep pose regression neural networks and clustered similarities. *IEEE Trans. Med. Imaging* **2020**, *39*, 3900–3909. [CrossRef]
66. Kim, I.; Misra, D.; Rodriguez, L.; Gill, M.; Liberton, D.K.; Almpani, K.; Lee, J.S.; Antani, S. Malocclusion classification on 3D cone-beam CT craniofacial images using multi-channel deep learning models. In Proceedings of the 2020 42nd Annual International Conference of the IEEE Engineering in Medicine & Biology Society (EMBC), Montreal, QC, Canada, 20–24 July 2020; pp. 1294–1298.
67. ter Horst, R.; van Weert, H.; Loonen, T.; Bergé, S.; Vinayahalingam, S.; Baan, F.; Maal, T.; de Jong, G.; Xi, T. Three-dimensional virtual planning in mandibular advancement surgery: Soft tissue prediction based on deep learning. *J. Craniomaxillofac. Surg.* **2021**, *49*, 775–782. [CrossRef]
68. Ma, Q.; Kobayashi, E.; Fan, B.; Hara, K.; Nakagawa, K.; Masamune, K.; Sakuma, I.; Suenaga, H. Machine-learning-based approach for predicting postoperative skeletal changes for orthognathic surgical planning. *Int. J. Med. Robot.* **2022**, *18*, e2379. [CrossRef]
69. Lin, H.H.; Chiang, W.C.; Yang, C.T.; Cheng, C.T.; Zhang, T.; Lo, L.J. On construction of transfer learning for facial symmetry assessment before and after orthognathic surgery. *Comput. Methods Programs Biomed.* **2021**, *200*, 105928. [CrossRef]
70. Nishiyama, M.; Ishibashi, K.; Ariji, Y.; Fukuda, M.; Nishiyama, W.; Umemura, M.; Katsumata, A.; Fujita, H.; Ariji, E. Performance of deep learning models constructed using panoramic radiographs from two hospitals to diagnose fractures of the mandibular condyle. *Dentomaxillofac. Radiol.* **2021**, *50*, 20200611. [CrossRef]
71. Krois, J.; Cantu, A.G.; Chaurasia, A.; Patil, R.; Chaudhari, P.K.; Gaudin, R.; Gehrung, S.; Schwendicke, F. Generalizability of deep learning models for dental image analysis. *Sci. Rep.* **2021**, *11*, 6102. [CrossRef]
72. Rischke, R.; Schneider, L.; Müller, K.; Samek, W.; Schwendicke, F.; Krois, J. Federated learning in dentistry: Chances and challenges. *J. Dent. Res.* **2022**, *101*, 1269–1273. [CrossRef]
73. Roy, S.; Meena, T.; Lim, S.J. Demystifying supervised learning in healthcare 4.0: A new reality of transforming diagnostic medicine. *Diagnostics* **2022**, *12*, 2549. [CrossRef]
74. Pfaehler, E.; Zhovannik, I.; Wei, L.; Boellaard, R.; Dekker, A.; Monshouwer, R.; El Naqa, I.; Bussink, J.; Gillies, R.; Wee, L.; et al. A systematic review and quality of reporting checklist for repeatability and reproducibility of radiomic features. *Phys. Imaging Radiat. Oncol.* **2021**, *20*, 69–75. [CrossRef] [PubMed]
75. Xue, C.; Yuan, J.; Lo, G.G.; Chang, A.T.Y.; Poon, D.M.C.; Wong, O.L.; Zhou, Y.; Chu, W.C.W. Radiomics feature reliability assessed by intraclass correlation coefficient: A systematic review. *Quant. Imaging Med. Surg.* **2021**, *11*, 4431–4460. [CrossRef] [PubMed]
76. Zhang, R.; Ai, Q.Y.H.; Wong, L.M.; Green, C.; Qamar, S.; So, T.Y.; Vlantis, A.C.; King, A.D. Radiomics for discriminating benign and malignant salivary gland tumors; which radiomic feature categories and MRI sequences should be used? *Cancers* **2022**, *14*, 5804. [CrossRef] [PubMed]
77. Wang, H.; Zhou, Y.; Wang, X.; Zhang, Y.; Ma, C.; Liu, B.; Kong, Q.; Yue, N.; Xu, Z.; Nie, K. Reproducibility and repeatability of CBCT-derived radiomics features. *Front. Oncol.* **2021**, *11*, 773512. [CrossRef]

78. Wong, L.M.; Ai, Q.Y.H.; Zhang, R.; Mo, F.; King, A.D. Radiomics for discrimination between early-stage nasopharyngeal carcinoma and benign hyperplasia with stable feature selection on MRI. *Cancers* **2022**, *14*, 3433. [CrossRef]
79. Bagher-Ebadian, H.; Siddiqui, F.; Liu, C.; Movsas, B.; Chetty, I.J. On the impact of smoothing and noise on robustness of CT and CBCT radiomics features for patients with head and neck cancers. *Med. Phys.* **2017**, *44*, 1755–1770. [CrossRef]
80. Sellami, S.; Bourbonne, V.; Hatt, M.; Tixier, F.; Bouzid, D.; Lucia, F.; Pradier, O.; Goasduff, G.; Visvikis, D.; Schick, U. Predicting response to radiotherapy of head and neck squamous cell carcinoma using radiomics from cone-beam CT images. *Acta Oncol.* **2022**, *61*, 73–80. [CrossRef]
81. Foy, J.J.; Robinson, K.R.; Li, H.; Giger, M.L.; Al-Hallaq, H.; Armato, S.G. Variation in algorithm implementation across radiomics software. *J. Med. Imaging (Bellingham)* **2018**, *5*, 044505. [CrossRef]
82. Bianchi, J.; Gonçalves, J.R.; Ruellas, A.C.O.; Vimort, J.B.; Yatabe, M.; Paniagua, B.; Hernandez, P.; Benavides, E.; Soki, F.N.; Cevidanes, L.H.S. Software comparison to analyze bone radiomics from high resolution CBCT scans of mandibular condyles. *Dentomaxillofac. Radiol.* **2019**, *48*, 20190049. [CrossRef]
83. Zwanenburg, A.; Vallières, M.; Abdalah, M.A.; Aerts, H.J.W.L.; Andrearczyk, V.; Apte, A.; Ashrafinia, S.; Bakas, S.; Beukinga, R.J.; Boellaard, R.; et al. The image biomarker standardization initiative: Standardized quantitative radiomics for high-throughput image-based phenotyping. *Radiology* **2020**, *295*, 328–338. [CrossRef]
84. Hung, K.F.; Yeung, A.W.K.; Bornstein, M.M.; Schwendicke, F. Personalized dental medicine, artificial intelligence, and their relevance for dentomaxillofacial imaging. *Dentomaxillofac. Radiol.* **2023**, *52*, 20220335. [CrossRef] [PubMed]

Disclaimer/Publisher's Note: The statements, opinions and data contained in all publications are solely those of the individual author(s) and contributor(s) and not of MDPI and/or the editor(s). MDPI and/or the editor(s) disclaim responsibility for any injury to people or property resulting from any ideas, methods, instructions or products referred to in the content.

diagnostics

MDPI

Article

CBCT Images to an STL Model: Exploring the "Critical Factors" to Binarization Thresholds in STL Data Creation

Takashi Kamio * and Taisuke Kawai

Department of Oral and Maxillofacial Radiology, School of Life Dentistry at Tokyo, The Nippon Dental University, 1-9-20 Fujimi, Chiyoda-ku, Tokyo 102-8159, Japan
* Correspondence: kamio@tky.ndu.ac.jp; Tel.: +81-3-3261-6516

Abstract: In-house fabrication of three-dimensional (3D) models for medical use has become easier in recent years. Cone beam computed tomography (CBCT) images are increasingly used as source data for fabricating osseous 3D models. The creation of a 3D CAD model begins with the segmentation of hard and soft tissues of the DICOM images and the creation of an STL model; however, it can be difficult to determine the binarization threshold in CBCT images. In this study, how the different CBCT scanning and imaging conditions of two different CBCT scanners affect the determination of the binarization threshold was evaluated. The key to efficient STL creation through voxel intensity distribution analysis was then explored. It was found that determination of the binarization threshold is easy for image datasets with a large number of voxels, sharp peak shapes, and narrow intensity distributions. Although the intensity distribution of voxels varied greatly among the image datasets, it was difficult to find correlations between different X-ray tube currents or image reconstruction filters that explained the differences. The objective observation of voxel intensity distribution may contribute to the determination of the binarization threshold for 3D model creation.

Keywords: cone beam computed tomography; imaging; radiology; oral and maxillofacial surgery; dentistry; DICOM; 3D printing; computer-aided design; STL data

1. Introduction

Recently, patient-specific three-dimensional (3D) models have been widely used in clinical practice. In particular, osseous 3D models are used to simulate surgical procedures on delicate anatomical structures during maxillofacial surgery, craniofacial surgery, and otolaryngology, and they are also used for surgical training and medical education. These 3D models allow users to actually manipulate the 3D model and view it from any angle. They can also be simulated with actual surgical instruments. Such an understanding of the three-dimensional anatomy of the surgical site contributes to a better understanding on the part of the surgeon, the surgical team, and medical students. This, in turn, is expected to lead to more predictable surgeries and shorter operating times. Its use as a preoperative educational tool for patients also contributes to better communication [1–4].

The generalization of 3D printing technologies has facilitated the fabrication of such 3D models from multi-detector row computed tomography (MDCT) images using desktop 3D printers; i.e., "one-stop 3D printing" [5].

Over the last two decades, cone beam computed tomography (CBCT), which has a smaller field of view (FOV) than MDCT and a higher spatial resolution, has become remarkably widespread, especially in the field of oral and maxillofacial surgery [6]. The design of osseous 3D models primarily requires 3D computer-aided design (CAD) data represented in stereolithography (STL) format. Although these data are used to create STL models (3D CAD models), the design of a more precise 3D model is expected to use image datasets from the CBCT scanner as the source of data.

The first step, binarization of the Digital Imaging and Communications in Medicine (DICOM) image dataset, is the most important operation in the sequence of fabricating

3D models. On the basis of numerous 3D model fabrication examples and our previous studies, unlike MDCT image datasets, it is sometimes difficult to determine the value to set the binarization threshold of an STL model using CBCT image datasets [7]. Several factors make the binarization of CBCT image datasets difficult. The biggest problem is that the threshold for binarization varies from one CBCT image dataset to another, and there is no specific value, such as a "CT value", for an MDCT image. The quality of image datasets exported as DICOM files varies from one CBCT unit to another, which is a major factor affecting the determination of the threshold value. These are also the problems that plague 3D CAD operators in determining the appropriate binarization threshold for creating STL models.

To enable anyone to create 3D models that satisfy clinical demands, it is necessary to establish a method to create highly precise 3D models from CBCT images in a reasonable procedure. It is also necessary to understand the characteristics of image datasets and what factors make it easy or difficult to determine the binarization threshold for STL model creation. Therefore, to understand the factors that affect the determination of the binarization threshold, this study aimed to evaluate the quality of STL models created from image datasets acquired with a CBCT scanner and to explore the factors relating to successful STL model creation from the perspective of 3D image engineering and 3D image processing.

2. Materials and Methods

2.1. Definition

In this study, DICOM image datasets exported to the STL file format (or data after segmentation) are called "STL data"; 3D surface CAD models (virtual 3D models) created from STL data are called "STL models". The model fabricated with a 3D printer from the STL data is referred to as a "3D model". The units for the intensity (brightness) values of the voxels are expressed in gray values (GV), according to a previous report by Katsumata et al. [8].

2.2. CBCT Scanning and Imaging to STL Model Creation

A dry human skull was used as a specimen. The skull was placed in a 20 cm cubic acrylic case filled with water and scanned. A cranial specimen with bilateral missing maxillary molars, without crown restorations, was used for maxillary alveolar and periapical maxillary sinus surgery (Figure 1). Scanning was performed with two different CBCT units, SOLIO XZ II (Asahi Roentgen Ind., Co. Ltd., Kyoto, Japan) and 3D Accuitomo F17 (J. Morita Mfg. Corp., Kyoto, Japan). After scanning, the image processing software attached to each CBCT unit was used to export the images as a DICOM file. Details of each scanning condition and the image reconstruction filters applied are shown in Table 1.

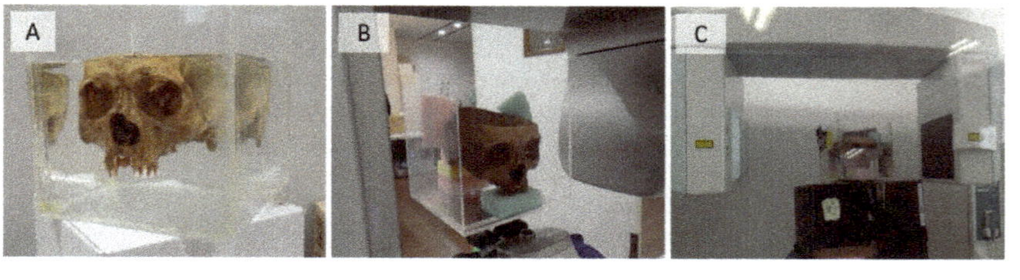

Figure 1. The specimen and CBCT units. (**A**) A specimen in an acrylic case filled with water, and the specimen in the (**B**) SOLIO XZ II (Asahi Roentgen Ind., Co. Ltd., Kyoto, Japan) scanner, and (**C**) 3D Accuitomo F17 (J. Morita Mfg. Corp., Kyoto, Japan) scanner.

Table 1. Overview of the scanning and image reconstruction filters for each CBCT unit and abbreviations for each DICOM image dataset.

CBCT Unit	X-ray Tube Voltage	Scanning Mode Field of View Voxel Size	Image Processing Software (Version)	X-ray Tube Current	Image Reconstruction Filter	Abbreviation
SOLIO XZ II	85 kV	I-MODE φ90 × 91 mm 0.177 mm	NEOPREMIUM2 (NeoExpCalc 1.0.17.0)	4.0 mA	Scattered ray correction	A4C
					Sharp	A4H
					Smooth	A4M
				6.0 mA	Scattered ray correction	A6C
					Sharp	A6H
					Smooth	A6M
				8.0 mA	Scattered ray correction	A8C
					Sharp	A8H
					Smooth	A8M
3D Accuitomo F17	85 kV	D140 × H100 Hi-Fi φ140 × 100 mm 0.200 mm	i-Dixel (3DXAPP 2.3.7.5)	4.0 mA	Bone	M4B
					Dental	M4D
					General	M4G
				6.0 mA	Bone	M6B
					Dental	M6D
					General	M6G
				8.0 mA	Bone	M8B
					Dental	M8D
					General	M8G

The impact of differences in the scanning X-ray tube current and image reconstruction filters on the determination of the binarization threshold in STL model creation was evaluated. The binarization threshold for each image was set so that both anterior and posterior nasal spines could be visualized and identified. Volume Extractor 3.0 (VE3, i-Plants Systems, Iwate, Japan), a 3D medical/general purpose image processing software package [9], was used to binarize the image datasets and create STL models. In VE3, the Marching Cube method was used as the isosurface extraction method. VE3 was used only for the conversion of image datasets to STL models, not for image linear interpolation or the noise reduction function. The removal of spatial polygonal noise (independent polygonal data not touching the surface of the STL model) was performed using the "Remove small polygons" command in the polygon data editing software package POLYGONALmeister ver7 (UEL Corp., Tokyo, Japan) [10].

2.3. Converting the DICOM Image Dataset to 256 Grayscale and Making a Histogram

ImageJ (version 1.53k, NIH, Bethesda, MD, USA) was used to convert the DICOM image dataset to 256 grayscale, and its histogram was used to evaluate the appearance of the voxel intensity distribution.

2.4. STL Model Superimposition, Comparison, and 3D Model Fabrication

To find the differences in the shape of each STL model created from the CBCT image dataset, the STL models were superimposed and the shape error (signed difference between two STL models) was observed. An STL model was created from the MDCT image dataset, which was used as the gold standard for the STL model shape. The MDCT scanner was an Aquilion 64 system (Canon Medical Systems Inc., Tochigi, Japan), with the following scanning conditions: X-ray tube voltage of 120 kV, X-ray tube current of 150 mA, slice thickness of 0.5 mm, FOV of 240 mm, a 512 × 512 matrix, and convolution kernel FC81 (bone sharp). The 3D evaluation software package spGauge 2014.1 (spG, ARMONICOS Co., Ltd., Shizuoka, Japan) was used for the superimposition of the created STL models and their color mapping. In the superimposition, one of the two STL models was moved using spG's best fit surface-based registration algorithm, and the operation was repeated until the misalignment with the other STL model was as close as possible to 0.00 mm. STL models created from CBCT image datasets were fabricated as 3D models using the same procedure as in our previous report [11].

3D model fabrication was performed with a desktop Fused Deposition Modeling (FDM) 3D printer (Value3D MagiX MF-800, Mutoh Industries, Tokyo, Japan). The 3D printing conditions are as follows: a PolyTerra-1.75 mm PLA filament, a laminating pitch of 0.2 mm, an infill density of 30%, a printing speed of 40 mm/s, and with support structures and rafts.

3. Results

3.1. Visibility of the Exported Images

Each image in the CBCT image dataset was imported and displayed in VE3, as shown in Figure 2. These are the native images with the default display settings of VE3. The same specimen was scanned; however, different X-ray tube currents and different applied image reconstruction filters resulted in different appearances.

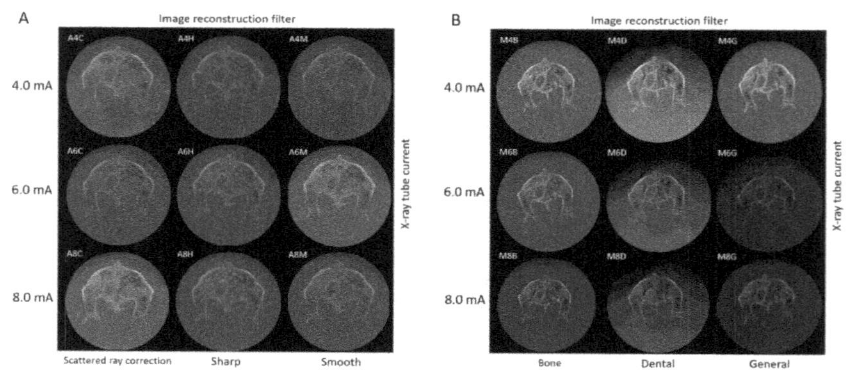

Figure 2. CBCT horizontal cross-sectional images of anterior and posterior nasal spines without window level setting displayed in Volume Extractor 3.0 using the (**A**) SOLIO XZ II scanner and (**B**) 3D Accuitomo F17 scanner.

3.2. Differences in the Shape of Each STL Model

The STL model created from each CBCT image dataset, with the binarization threshold for STL model creation set to the GV where the anterior and posterior nasal spines can be identified, is shown in Figure 3. For each image dataset, there was a difference in the shape of the STL model and the number of polygons that were mixed in as noise.

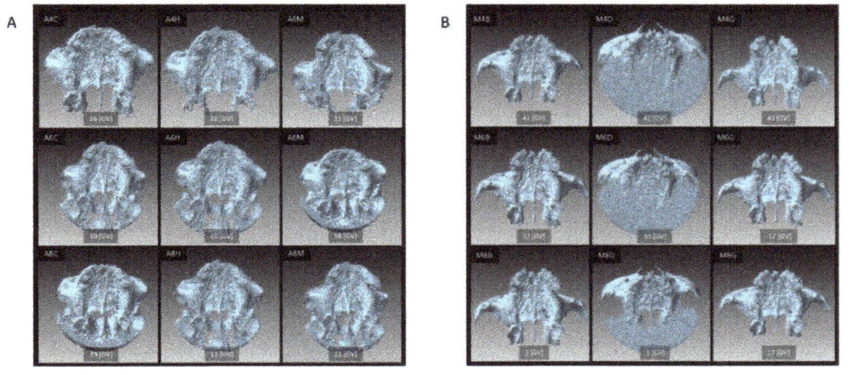

Figure 3. The STL models from the (**A**) SOLIO XZ II scanner and (**B**) 3D Accuitomo F17 scanner were created with the binarization threshold set to an arbitrary value. The abbreviation of each STL model is shown at the left shoulder of each figure, and the binarization threshold is shown at the bottom center of each figure. The GV indicates the percentile after the intensity value of each image dataset was converted to 256 grayscale.

3.3. Histogram of the Voxel Intensity Distribution

Figure 4A,B show the voxel intensity distribution of each CBCT image dataset, and Figure 4C shows the voxel intensity distribution of the MDCT image dataset used as the gold standard for STL model creation. In both CBCT image datasets, each voxel had a single peak; however, the maximum value and range of the peak varied. Histogram observations showed that, compared with the 3D Accuitomo F17, the SOLIO XZ II had fewer maximum voxels and tended to converge at the center of the voxel intensity value distribution. In the image dataset acquired on the Aquilion 64, the distribution of the voxel intensity values was bimodal, with apex-like peaks and narrow ranges.

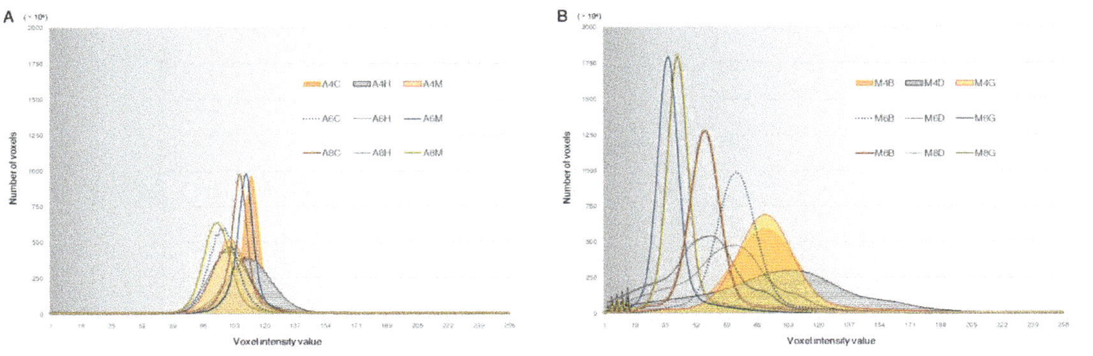

Figure 4. *Cont.*

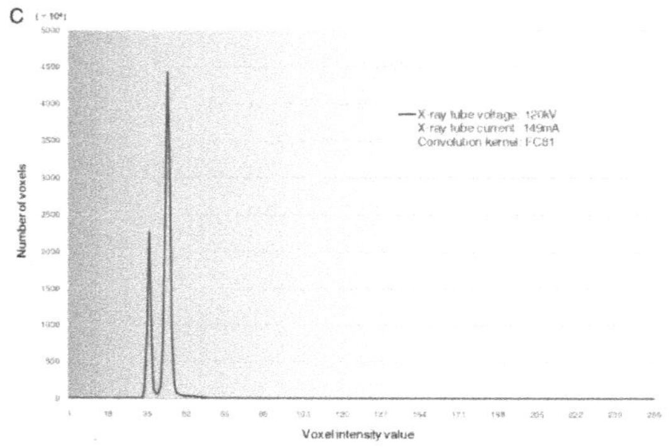

Figure 4. Histograms of voxel intensity for CBCT images from the (**A**) SOLIO XZ II and (**B**) 3D Accuitomo F17 scanners and (**C**) Aquilion 64 MDCT scanner images. The vertical axis represents the number of voxels and the horizontal axis represents the voxel intensity value in 256 grayscale.

3.4. Differences in Images for Each GV

The image visibility also differed significantly depending on the binarization threshold. At lower threshold values, the spatial noise increased. However, a higher threshold resulted in less replicability of thin areas of bone tissue (Figure 5).

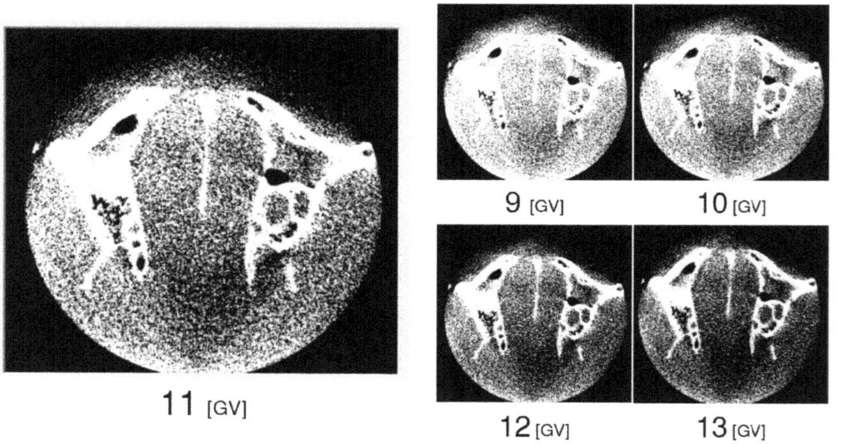

Figure 5. Images at different binarization threshold values (image dataset: A4C). The gray values shown at the bottom of each figure are the native voxel values of the CBCT image (in this case, from 3721 to −2359 [GV]) converted to 256 grayscale.

3.5. Shape Error of the STL Models

The superimposed shape error of the STL models created from the two CBCT and MDCT image datasets, respectively, showed that both the SOLIO XZ II and 3D Accuitomo F17 had more noise in the teeth and surrounding tissue, and the error was large. Additionally, the SOLIO XZ II had a rougher surface than the 3D Accuitomo F17, with a higher percentage of green to yellow or slightly distended areas (Figure 6).

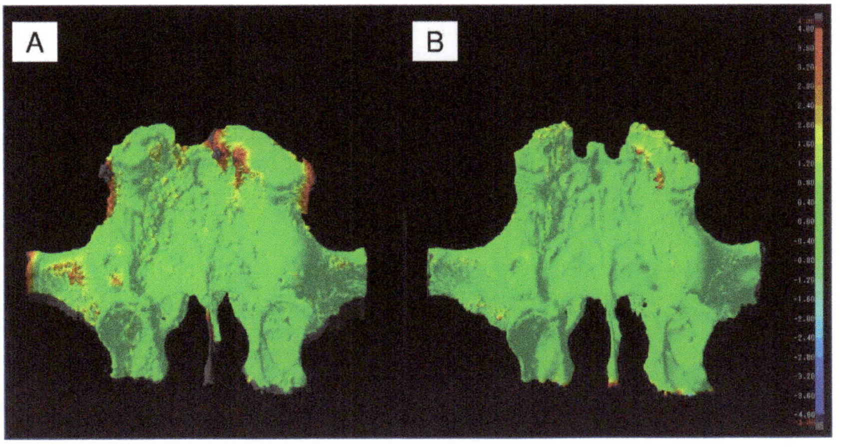

Figure 6. Shape error of two superimposed STL models. (**A**) CBCT STL model (image dataset: A4C) vs. MDCT STL model. (**B**) CBCT STL model (image dataset: M8G) vs. MDCT STL model. The areas where shape errors compared with the MDCT STL model used as the gold standard were observed are in color. Positive errors (expansion) are shown in warm colors and negative errors (contraction) are shown in cool colors.

4. Discussion

Dental implant surgeries, such as maxillary sinus floor augmentation, and maxillofacial surgery, such as a Le Fort I osteotomy, require delicate handling of the maxillary alveolar bone, maxillary sinus, and sphenoid process regions. As a result, highly precise 3D models are necessary for their simulation. In this study, we explored the optimal binarization threshold for STL model creation to fabricate osseous 3D models that faithfully replicate delicate and complicated anatomical structures.

Two flagship CBCT scanners from two different suppliers were used. One is the SOLIO XZ II, a multifunctional scanner capable of CBCT scanning and panoramic imaging. This scanner is mainly used in the field of dentistry and maxillofacial surgery. The other is the 3D Accuitomo F17 scanner, which is a dedicated scanning unit for CBCT, with a range from a minimum φ40 mm × height of 40 mm to a maximum of φ170 mm to a height of 230 mm, and 11 different FOVs can be selected according to the region of interest. The Accuitomo F17 scanner is primarily used in the fields of oral and maxillofacial surgery, craniofacial surgery, and otolaryngology.

Three steps are required to create a 3D model from an image dataset [6,11]. The first step is to acquire the 3D volumetric data of the object as a DICOM file. The second step is to segment the anatomical structures of the 3D model fabrication object from the surrounding structures and export them to a 3D CAD model in STL file format. While segmentation of hard and soft tissues is relatively easy, the subsequent STL model creation is sometimes difficult for two reasons. Small or thin bones (such as in the maxillary sinus, nasal cavity, or orbital floor) and narrow bone cavities (such as the joint cavity of the temporomandibular joint) are not easily reflected in the STL model. Problems resulting from the scanning characteristics of CBCT/MDCT (e.g., metallic artifacts from dental materials, beam hardening, overshooting, and undershooting) reduce image visibility and make it difficult to determine the threshold for binarization. The final step is to generate data for 3D printing, called G-code, from the created STL model and run the 3D printer. Failure in any of these steps results in poor quality of the 3D model. Therefore, the creation of satisfactory STL data is the most important operation in the sequence of 3D model fabrication [6,12].

CBCT images do not contain the quantitative physical quantities that are in MDCT images, such as "CT values" or "Hounsfield units" [13–15]. In other words, because the GV of a CBCT image is not a linearized value, the binarization threshold is also difficult to determine using standard methodologies. Therefore, the shape of the STL model may be highly dependent on the discretion of the 3D CAD operator. The 3D model created from the STL model (A6M), which the authors created by determining the binarization threshold, is shown in Figure 7. Even with the full use of polygon data editing software packages, it was difficult to control the noisy 3D CAD model. The detail of the fabricated 3D model is somewhat less replicable, with numerous irregular structures appearing on the surface.

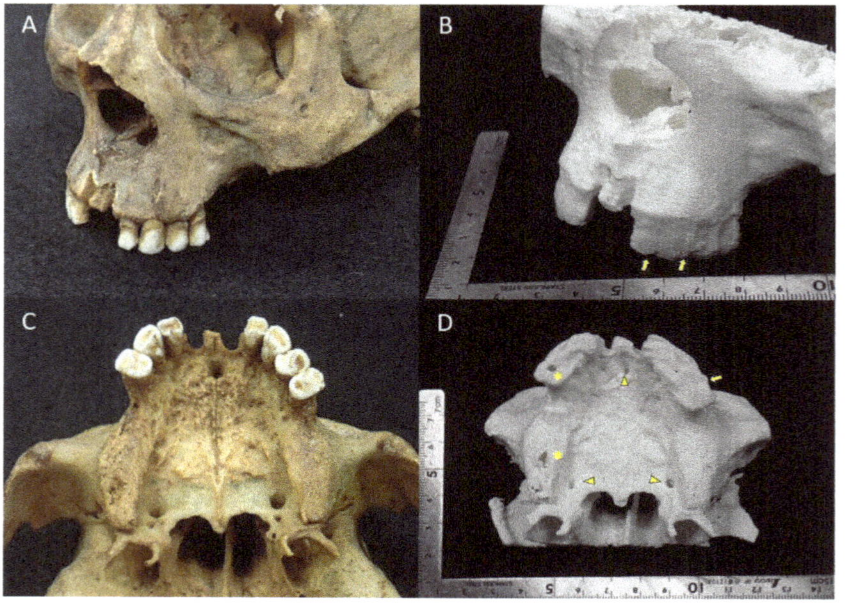

Figure 7. (**A**,**C**) Close-up view of the specimen. (**B**,**D**) Close-up view of the 3D model fabricated from an STL model (image dataset: A4C) with a desktop FDM 3D printer. In fabricating the 3D model, the STL model was smoothed, noise-reduced, and polygon-count-reduced using POLYGONALmeister Ver 7. Observations of the 3D model show that the replication of the teeth and surrounding tissues is poor (arrows). The incisal and greater palatine foramen are also generally narrower (arrowheads). Partial defects on the surface of the 3D model because of 3D printing errors are noted (*).

With our approach, differences in the visibility of each X-ray tube current and image reconstruction filter—that is, differences in the scanning and imaging characteristics of each CBCT unit—could be objectively visualized as differences in the intensity distribution of voxels. This is the same as a visualization of the differences in image contrast in each image dataset. These differences in image datasets can be attributed to differences in the method of image reconstruction performed by image processing software after CBCT image data acquisition; i.e., differences in the image gamma correction applied to each filter. It was easier to determine the binarization threshold of an image dataset with high image contrast that was made in the histogram as a positive curve with more voxels, high peaks, a relatively narrow distribution, and a steep slope. Unsuitable binarization thresholds can result in poor replication of details in the STL model. 3D models from poor-quality STL models can, for example, lead to unintended defects or cavities, thus compromising the reliability of the surgical simulation. This result partly explains why it is difficult to determine the binarization threshold when the peak number of voxels is too low or the voxel intensity distribution range is too narrow or too wide. Although the binarization threshold required for STL data depends on the application of the 3D model and cannot be uniformly specified, a histogram of the voxel intensity distribution of the image dataset would help determine the binarization threshold for creating STL models that satisfy clinical demand.

There are numerous reports on automatic segmentation of CBCT and MDCT images. However, even for MDCT images, for which voxel intensity values can be obtained quantitatively, automatic segmentation is difficult to perform. For CBCT images, however, there are many different scanners available, with varying scanning and imaging characteristics, making segmentation a very difficult challenge [16–22]. Furthermore, to our knowledge, there are few reports evaluating MDCT images for STL data creation for 3D model fabrication, and there are no reports using the same approach as ours using CBCT images [23–26]. CBCT scanners are expected to be used as 3D scanning devices for dental casts and dental prosthetics (surgical guides, dentures) [27–29]. As the demand for 3D printed models increases, better STL data are needed and their importance will increase. Because the two CBCT units used in this study were not equipped with image reconstruction filters that are specialized for the 3D model, such as the "STL data creation mode", the binarization threshold for creating STL data had to be determined manually by the 3D CAD operators. Considering the rapid development of 3D technology, a CBCT unit equipped with an "Imaging filter for 3D copy" that can create optimal STL data under optimal scanning and imaging conditions will likely be available soon.

A limitation of this study is that there were only 18 image datasets with each scanning X-ray tube voltage set to 85 kV and three representative image reconstruction filters. Both CBCT units had other scanning modes. In addition to the scanning conditions, such as the X-ray tube voltage and tube current, it is possible to select a larger or smaller FOV according to the object size and image reconstruction filters according to the diagnostic purpose. Another limitation is that there is no standard for determining the binarization threshold for creating STL models from CBCT images. We have used a threshold where the targeted anatomical structures are somewhat visible. However, we recognize that this binarization threshold value was determined by the experience of the authors, who are also 3D CAD/3D printing operators, and it is lacking objectivity. There is currently no methodology to prove this binarization threshold is appropriate; however, that is a topic for future research.

In this study, we evaluated voxel intensity distribution histograms made from DICOM image datasets from two different CBCT scanners to determine why it is difficult to create STL data for a 3D model from CBCT images and how to address this issue. The image appearance varied greatly depending on the scanning and imaging conditions, and the binarization threshold also varied relative to each image.

In conclusion, the results of this study suggest the importance of understanding the scanning and imaging characteristics of each CBCT device in advance to determine the optimal and objective binarization threshold. Our approach, which enables facile observation of the visibility of the voxel intensity distribution and is technically simple, may help find the "critical factors" to binarization threshold determination, which is essential for the fabrication of 3D models for the medical field.

Author Contributions: Conceptualization, T.K. (Taisuke Kawai); methodology, T.K. (Taisuke Kawai); software, T.K. (Takashi Kamio); validation, T.K. (Takashi Kamio); formal analysis, T.K. (Takashi Kamio); investigation, T.K. (Taisuke Kawai) and T.K. (Takashi Kamio); resources, T.K. (Taisuke Kawai); data curation, T.K. (Takashi Kamio); writing—original draft preparation, T.K. (Takashi Kamio); writing—review and editing, T.K. (Taisuke Kawai); visualization, T.K. (Takashi Kamio); supervision, T.K. (Taisuke Kawai); project administration, T.K. (Taisuke Kawai); funding acquisition, T.K. (Taisuke Kawai) All authors have read and agreed to the published version of the manuscript.

Funding: This research received no external funding.

Institutional Review Board Statement: Not applicable.

Informed Consent Statement: Not applicable.

Data Availability Statement: The data presented in this study are available on request from the corresponding author. The data are not publicly available because they belong to an academic institution.

Acknowledgments: We would like to thank Asahi Roentgen Ind., Co. Ltd., and J. Morita Mfg. Corp. for their substantial cooperation on this study.

Conflicts of Interest: The authors declare no conflict of interest.

References

1. Tack, P.; Victor, J.; Gemmel, P.; Annemans, L. 3D-printing techniques in a medical setting: A systematic literature review. *Biomed. Eng. Online* **2016**, *15*, 115. [CrossRef] [PubMed]
2. Zheng, B.; Wang, X.; Zheng, Y.; Feng, J. 3D-printed model improves clinical assessment of surgeons on anatomy. *J. Robot Surg.* **2019**, *3*, 61–67. [CrossRef] [PubMed]
3. Narita, M.; Takaki, T.; Shibahara, T.; Iwamoto, M.; Yakushiji, T.; Kamio, T. Utilization of desktop 3D printer-fabricated "Cost-Effective" 3D models in orthognathic surgery. *Maxillofac. Plast. Reconstr. Surg.* **2020**, *42*, 24. [CrossRef] [PubMed]
4. Tomohisa, O.; Kamio, T.; Maeda, Y.; Tsubosaki, K.; Kato, T.; Iwata, H. Application of Medical Imaging and 3D Printing Technology in Teaching the Handling of Novel Medicine in Periodontal Surgery. *Cureus* **2022**, *14*, e29271. [CrossRef]
5. Kamio, T.; Hayashi, K.; Onda, T.; Takaki, T.; Shibahara, T.; Yakushiji, T.; Shibui, T.; Kato, H. Utilizing a low-cost desktop 3D printer to develop a "one-stop 3D printing lab" for oral and maxillofacial surgery and dentistry fields. *3D Print Med.* **2018**, *4*, 6. [CrossRef] [PubMed]
6. Arai, Y.; Tammisalo, E.; Iwai, K.; Hashimoto, K.; Shinoda, K. Development of a compact computed tomographic apparatus for dental use. *Dentomaxillofac. Radiol.* **1999**, *28*, 245–248. [CrossRef] [PubMed]
7. Kamio, T.; Suzuki, M.; Asaumi, R.; Kawai, T. DICOM segmentation and STL creation for 3D printing: A process and software package comparison for osseous anatomy. *3D Print Med.* **2020**, *6*, 17. [CrossRef]
8. Katsumata, A.; Hirukawa, A.; Okumura, S.; Naitoh, M.; Fujishita, M.; Ariji, E.; Langlais, R.P. Effects of image artifacts on gray-value density in limited-volume cone-beam computerized tomography. *Oral Surg. Oral Med. Oral Pathol. Oral Radiol. Endod.* **2007**, *104*, 829–836. [CrossRef]
9. Doi, A.; Suzuki, S.; Yamasa, F.; Itoh, F.; Matsui, K.; Sachio, M.; Itoh, S. Volume Extractor Ver.3.0- 3D Image Processing and 3D Model Reconstruction. *IIEE J.* **2008**, *37*, 1037–1043.
10. Tanimoto, S. Collaborative research on polygon engineering with RIKEN. *Unisys Technol. Rev.* **2012**, *32*, 283–292. (In Japanese). Available online: https://pr.biprogy.com/tec_info/tr114/11413.pdf (accessed on 19 January 2023).
11. Kamio, T.; Onda, T. Fused Deposition Modeling 3D Printing in Oral and Maxillofacial Surgery: Problems and Solutions. *Cureus* **2022**, *14*, e28906. [CrossRef] [PubMed]
12. Adolphs, N.; Liu, W.; Keeve, E.; Hoffmeister, B. Craniomaxillofacial surgery planning based on 3D models derived from Cone-Beam CT data. *Comput. Aided Surg.* **2013**, *18*, 101–108. [CrossRef] [PubMed]
13. Rong, Y.; Smilowitz, J.; Tewatia, D.; Tome, W.A.; Paliwal, B. Dose calculation on kV cone beam CT images: An investigation of the Hu-density conversion stability and dose accuracy using the site-specific calibration. *Med. Dosim.* **2010**, *35*, 195–207. [CrossRef] [PubMed]
14. Molteni, R. Prospects and challenges of rendering tissue density in Hounsfield units for cone beam computed tomography. *Oral Surg. Oral Med. Oral Pathol. Oral Radiol.* **2013**, *116*, 105–119. [CrossRef] [PubMed]
15. Pauwels, R.; Jacobs, R.; Singer, S.R.; Mupparapu, M. CBCT-based bone quality assessment: Are Hounsfield units applicable? *Dentomaxillofac. Radiol.* **2015**, *44*, 20140238. [CrossRef]
16. Pauwels, R.; Araki, K.; Siewerdsen, J.H.; Thongvigitmanee, S.S. Technical aspects of dental CBCT: State of the art. *Dentomaxillofac. Radiol.* **2015**, *44*, 20140224. [CrossRef] [PubMed]
17. Ronkainen, A.P.; Al-Gburi, A.; Liimatainen, T.; Matikka, H. A dose-neutral image quality comparison of different CBCT and CT systems using paranasal sinus imaging protocols and phantoms. *Eur. Arch. Otorhinolaryngol.* **2022**, *279*, 4407–4414. [CrossRef] [PubMed]
18. Jin, J.Y.; Ren, L.; Liu, Q.; Kim, J.; Wen, N.; Guan, H.; Movsas, B.; Chetty, I.J. Combining scatter reduction and correction to improve image quality in cone-beam computed tomography (CBCT). *Med. Phys.* **2010**, *37*, 5634–5644. [CrossRef]
19. Zheng, J.; Zhang, D.; Huang, K.; Sun, Y. A CBCT series slice image segmentation method. *J. Xray. Sci. Technol.* **2018**, *26*, 815–832. [CrossRef]
20. Wang, L.; Li, J.P.; Ge, Z.P.; Li, G. CBCT image based segmentation method for tooth pulp cavity region extraction. *Dentomaxillofac. Radiol.* **2019**, *48*, 20180236. [CrossRef]
21. Li, C.; Lin, L.; Zheng, Z.; Chung, C.H. A User-Friendly Protocol for Mandibular Segmentation of CBCT Images for Superimposition and Internal Structure Analysis. *J. Clin. Med.* **2021**, *10*, 127. [CrossRef] [PubMed]
22. Borohovitz, C.L.; Abraham, Z.; Redmond, W.R. The diagnostic advantage of a CBCT-derived segmented STL rendition of the teeth and jaws using an AI algorithm. *J. Clin. Orthod.* **2021**, *55*, 361–369. [PubMed]

23. Lo Giudice, A.; Ronsivalle, V.; Grippaudo, C.; Lucchese, A.; Muraglie, S.; Lagravère, M.O.; Isola, G. One Step before 3D Printing—Evaluation of Imaging Software Accuracy for 3-Dimensional Analysis of the Mandible: A Comparative Study Using a Surface-to-Surface Matching Technique. *Materials* **2020**, *13*, 2798. [CrossRef] [PubMed]
24. van Eijnatten, M.; Koivisto, J.; Karhu, K.; Forouzanfar, T.; Wolff, J. The impact of manual threshold selection in medical additive manufacturing. *Int. J. Comput. Assist. Radiol. Surg.* **2017**, *12*, 607–615. [CrossRef]
25. van Eijnatten, M.; Berger, F.H.; de Graaf, P.; Koivisto, J.; Forouzanfar, T.; Wolff, J. Influence of CT parameters on STL model accuracy. *Rapid Prototyp. J.* **2017**, *23*, 678–685. [CrossRef]
26. Wu, A.M.; Shao, Z.X.; Wang, J.S.; Yang, X.D.; Weng, W.Q.; Wang, X.Y.; Xu, H.Z.; Chi, Y.L.; Lin, Z.K. The accuracy of a method for printing three-dimensional spinal models. *PLoS ONE* **2015**, *10*, e0124291. [CrossRef]
27. Rangel, F.A.; Maal, T.J.; Bronkhorst, E.M.; Breuning, K.H.; Schols, J.G.; Bergé, S.J.; Kuijpers-Jagtman, A.M. Accuracy and reliability of a novel method for fusion of digital dental casts and Cone Beam Computed Tomography scans. *PLoS ONE* **2013**, *8*, e59130. [CrossRef]
28. Kane, B.; Shah, K.C. A dual scan approach to creating an accurate dental surface for virtual implant planning: A dental technique. *J. Prosthet. Dent.* **2021**, *126*, 464–470. [CrossRef]
29. Michelinakis, G.; Apostolakis, D.; Pavlakis, E.; Kourakis, G.; Papavasiliou, G. Accuracy of IOS in Full-Arch Dentate Patients Compared to CBCT Cast-Scanning. An In-Vivo Study. *Eur. J. Prosthodont. Restor. Dent.* **2019**, *27*, 122–130.

Disclaimer/Publisher's Note: The statements, opinions and data contained in all publications are solely those of the individual author(s) and contributor(s) and not of MDPI and/or the editor(s). MDPI and/or the editor(s) disclaim responsibility for any injury to people or property resulting from any ideas, methods, instructions or products referred to in the content.

diagnostics

MDPI

Review

CBCT for Diagnostics, Treatment Planning and Monitoring of Sinus Floor Elevation Procedures

Nermin Morgan [1,2,*], Jan Meeus [3], Sohaib Shujaat [1,3,4], Simone Cortellini [5,6], Michael M. Bornstein [7] and Reinhilde Jacobs [1,3,8]

1 OMFS IMPATH Research Group, Department of Imaging & Pathology, Faculty of Medicine, KU Leuven, 3000 Leuven, Belgium
2 Department of Oral Medicine, Faculty of Dentistry, Mansoura University, Mansoura 35516, Egypt
3 Department of Oral and Maxillofacial Surgery, University Hospitals Leuven, Campus Sint-Rafael, 3000 Leuven, Belgium
4 King Abdullah International Medical Research Center, Department of Maxillofacial Surgery and Diagnostic Sciences, College of Dentistry, King Saud bin Abdulaziz University for Health Sciences, Ministry of National Guard Health Affairs, Riyadh 11426, Saudi Arabia
5 Department of Oral Health Sciences, Section of Periodontology, KU Leuven, 3000 Leuven, Belgium
6 Department of Dentistry, University Hospitals Leuven, KU Leuven, 3000 Leuven, Belgium
7 Department of Oral Health & Medicine, University Center for Dental Medicine Basel UZB, University of Basel, 4058 Basel, Switzerland
8 Department of Dental Medicine, Karolinska Institute, 141 04 Huddinge, Sweden
* Correspondence: nermin.morgan@student.kuleuven.be

Abstract: Sinus floor elevation (SFE) is a standard surgical technique used to compensate for alveolar bone resorption in the posterior maxilla. Such a surgical procedure requires radiographic imaging pre- and postoperatively for diagnosis, treatment planning, and outcome assessment. Cone beam computed tomography (CBCT) has become a well-established imaging modality in the dentomaxillofacial region. The following narrative review is aimed to provide clinicians with an overview of the role of three-dimensional (3D) CBCT imaging for diagnostics, treatment planning, and postoperative monitoring of SFE procedures. CBCT imaging prior to SFE provides surgeons with a more detailed view of the surgical site, allows for the detection of potential pathologies three-dimensionally, and helps to virtually plan the procedure more precisely while reducing patient morbidity. In addition, it serves as a useful follow-up tool for assessing sinus and bone graft changes. Meanwhile, using CBCT imaging has to be standardized and justified based on the recognized diagnostic imaging guidelines, taking into account both the technical and clinical considerations. Future studies are recommended to incorporate artificial intelligence-based solutions for automating and standardizing the diagnostic and decision-making process in the context of SFE procedures to further improve the standards of patient care.

Keywords: CBCT; three-dimensional imaging; maxillary sinus; sinus floor elevation; sinus floor augmentation

1. Introduction

Alveolar bone atrophy in the maxillary posterior region is inevitable following tooth extraction, resulting in horizontal and vertical ridge resorption [1,2]. If a dental implant is inserted in bone having inadequate volume, there is a high risk of compromised implant stability and poor prognosis [3,4]. In order to compensate for reduced bone height and volume of the maxillary posterior region, sinus floor elevation (SFE) is performed for bone reconstruction. It involves lifting up of the Schneiderian membrane, which is usually followed by the placement of a bone graft [5–9].

The two main techniques for SFE are either a direct approach using a lateral window or indirect with the transalveolar technique. In the lateral window approach, an osteotomy is performed in the buccal wall of the maxilla, creating access through the lateral bone wall of the sinus cavity [10–12]. The transalveolar technique is a less invasive technique that was modified by Summers [13], where a transcrestal osteotome is applied to elevate the sinus floor, pushing bone substitutes beyond the level of the original sinus floor [14]. This technique has been recommended in areas with sufficient alveolar crest width and where a residual vertical bone height of $\geq$5 mm is available [15]. In cases where the alveolar bone height is less than 5 mm, the lateral window approach is recommended [16].

To date, various graft materials have been successfully used for SFE solely or in combination with each other [17], such as autograft [18–21] (intraoral: chin, retromolar region, mandibular ramus, maxillary tuberosity [22,23]; extraoral: iliac crest, fibula, tibia [24–26]), allograft [27–29] (fresh, frozen, freeze-dried bone [30,31]), xenograft [32–36] (deproteinized bovine bone [37–39]), and phytogenic material [39–41] (Gusuibu, coral-based bone substitutes, and marine algae).

Along with patient history and clinical examination, radiographic examination is an essential component of preliminary diagnostics, treatment planning, and outcome assessment in patients requiring SFE. Previously, two-dimensional (2D) panoramic radiography acted as a clinical standard. However, it suffers from certain inherent limitations, which can negatively impact the task at hand, such as magnification, distortion, and superimposition [16,42].

Three-dimensional (3D) preoperative imaging of the specific site of augmentation becomes a prerequisite in order to provide needed information about the morphologic characteristics and/or pathological conditions of the sinus and residual ridge [43–45]. Some studies have used computed tomography (CT) for the planning of sinus grafting [46] and precalculated the augmented bone volume needed [47–50]. However, the use of CT imaging is limited for most dental practitioners due to the high costs, large size of the device, and high radiation dose. To overcome these general limitations, 3D imaging in the form of cone beam CT (CBCT) has become a standard [43,44] for patients requiring maxillary sinus procedures. Recently, various CBCT imaging systems with low-dose protocols have also been made commercially available, which are not only affordable and compact to be used in a private dental practice but also provide 3D imaging with a lower radiation dose exposure to the patient [51,52].

The aim of the present review was to discuss the role of CBCT imaging for diagnostics, treatment planning, and postoperative monitoring of SFE as well as recommend future research directions, which could be useful for improving the current standard of patient care.

2. Use of CBCT for Diagnostics and Treatment Planning Prior to SFE

CBCT has been widely employed for diagnosis and preoperative treatment planning in all fields of dentistry [53], allowing for 3D visualization of dental structures and multiplanar reconstruction. It can provide cross-sectional images of the alveolar bone with the ability to accurately measure its height, width, and depict surrounding vital structures, such as the maxillary sinus. It allows for thorough assessment of the bone quality (density) and quantity (thickness) as well as the detection of bony changes, such as fractures or malformations. Furthermore, CBCT can be used for volume quantification that could help monitor bone remodeling and sinus disease [45,53,54].

Based on the recommendations of the American Academy of Oral and Maxillofacial Radiology (AAOMR) [55], CBCT imaging prior to SFE provides surgeons with a more detailed view of the surgical site. This helps to plan the surgical intervention more precisely while reducing patient morbidity. Additionally, it can be used to detect any potential problems and/or present pathology in advance, allowing for a safer and more successful bone grafting procedure. This also comes in accordance with the consideration of sinus augmentation mentioned in the updated guidelines for the use of diagnostic imaging in implant dentistry published by the European Association for Osseointegration (E.A.O.) [56].

From a technical point of view, in patients requiring CBCT acquisition for diagnostics, the "as low as reasonably achievable" (ALARA) principle has gone through a long history of evolution. Recently, some expert opinions advocated to rename it to "as low as diagnostically acceptable" (ALADA) [57] and, more recently, "as low as diagnostically acceptable being indication-oriented and patient-specific" (ALADAIP) [58]. These up to date principles highlight the need for actually optimizing rather than simply minimizing doses, taking into account not only the diagnosis but also treatment planning such as preoperative sinus grafting. For instance, when there is evidence of sinus pathology or sinus drainage is expected to be impaired, which might jeopardize the SFE outcomes, it is justifiable to extend the field of view (FOV) to include the whole of the maxillary sinus, including the ostio-meatal complex [59–62].

Furthermore, a multitude of CBCT devices exist in the market with variable scanning parameters, which include slice thickness, FOV, mAs, kVp, and scan time [63]. All these factors influence the image quality and amount of administered radiation dose. Generally, the effective radiation doses of CBCT devices for maxillofacial applications should preferably be 20 to 100 μSv; however, the doses of commercially available devices range from 10 to 1000 μSv depending on the parameter's settings. Nevertheless, it is still lower than that of CT devices, which might vary between 474 and 1160 μSv [45,64]. Saying that, it is recommended to justify and optimize CBCT acquisition parameters for diagnostic tasks in an attempt to decrease the risk of high radiation dose exposure to the patient.

From a clinical point of view, CBCT enhances the diagnostic evaluation relative to 2D imaging by providing additional information related to the maxillary sinuses and surrounding structures. This diagnostic information could be a useful adjunct for SFE planning, as a thorough radiological assessment is not only important for the sinus surgery but also for implant placement. The diagnostic features extracted from CBCT images that could be clinically relevant for performing a successful SFE procedure, which could very well remain undetected with 2D imaging, are as follows:

- *Anatomy of maxillary sinus and alveolar ridge*

CBCT imaging provides detailed anatomical information related to sinus anatomy. These findings allow the surgeon to assess the sinus morphology, density, and volume of the residual alveolar ridge, which might in turn help to determine the best approach for accessing the sinus and to evaluate the suitability of the patient's bone for grafting [55,65].

- *Relation of maxillary sinus to the roots of adjacent teeth*

If there is an intimate contact between the root(s) of the teeth and the Schneiderian membrane, the risk of membrane perforation during the sinus lift procedure is increased. Hence, it is important to evaluate the root proximity to the sinus during the diagnostic phase through CBCT imaging for decreasing the risk of perforation [66,67]. Additionally, the health state of adjacent teeth should be examined for the presence of pre-existing apical pathology that could result in sinus graft infection [68].

- *Thickness of the Schneiderian membrane*

CBCT has been reported to be a useful tool for assessing the thickness of the Schneiderian membrane [60,69], which has also been reported to be associated with the occurrence of membrane perforation [70]. Healthy sinus mucosa has a mean thickness of 1 mm, although there is a wide range of variability among individuals [71]. Meanwhile, it should be noted that the risk of sinusitis following SFE increases when the membrane thickness is over 2 mm [72], and a higher risk of ostium obstruction exists if the membrane thickness is over 5 mm [73].

- *Maxillary sinus septum* [74,75]

Prior evidence suggests that at least one-third of patients have sinus septa, which are visualized ideally through 3D imaging [76]. The knowledge about septa location and morphology is a key factor in planning SFE, as it is associated with an increased risk of sinus membrane perforation during the procedure. Furthermore, if present, the osteotomy design might also require an alteration from a single window technique to two smaller windows on either side of the maxillary sinus floor septum or the use of a W-shaped trapdoor technique. Hence, CBCT imaging is the key to success in devising a proper treatment plan [77].

- *Maxillary sinus ostium*

Sinus healing following SFE is largely dependent on sufficient drainage of the nasal cavity. If the ostium is not patent, the drainage would be impaired, which could cause sinusitis or surgical failure [72]. For guaranteeing appropriate mucociliary drainage and clearance, the ostium patency must be evaluated prior to surgery. In addition, the sinus should be assessed for the presence of accessory ostia, which can interfere with sinus ventilation and drainage [78].

- *Maxillary sinus floor width*

The distance and angulation between the lateral and medial maxillary sinus walls are also important anatomical features to be evaluated with CBCT imaging. It allows determining the difficulty level of performing SFE, as too narrow or too large sinuses with sharp angulations are considered complex cases. Moreover, accurate measurement of the sinus width based on CBCT imaging is also crucial for deciding the surgical approach; for example, a trapdoor SFE technique is contraindicated in patients having narrow sinuses [79].

- *Thickness of the lateral maxillary sinus wall*

Maxillary sinus lateral wall thickness is an important parameter to be assessed using CBCT imaging at the diagnostic stage because SFE through a thick wall is difficult to perform, takes longer time and is more prone to perforation. Hence, CBCT imaging is suggested to help with the decision-making process, as it allows the surgeon to 3D evaluate the sinus wall and select the region with the least thickness to avoid complications [80].

- *Alveolar antral artery*

CBCT imaging allows a clear depiction of the antral artery, allowing for an optimal planning of the surgical access to the sinus. Alveolar antral arteries with a diameter more than 0.5 mm can be observed on CBCT, and profuse bleeding should be expected if the artery has a diameter more than 3 mm [81]. If present at the osteotomy site, the use of a piezosurgery device is preferred. Moreover, changing the osteotomy window design from an oval to a round shape through either above or below this artery could avoid injury [82].

- *Estimation of graft volume*

Using the combination of CBCT images along with the various planning software systems available allows for measuring and extracting the sinus volume necessary to be grafted [83]. Adequate preoperative planning of the graft volume may help to avoid sinus over-filling and potentially occluding the ostium, decide on the ratio of bone and bone substitutes to be mixed, and estimate the cost of xenografts prior to the actual operation [47,48]. It is worth noting that in cases where an autogenous graft will be harvested, preoperative knowledge of the amount of graft required is useful in selecting the optimal donor region, reducing the time and complexity of the surgical procedures, as well as minimizing potential postoperative complications [84].

- *Incidental findings*

The role of CBCT in revealing incidental findings (IFs) which are not related to the primary scan indication also cannot be ignored. Several studies have reported a high prevalence of IFs in the maxillary sinus region on CBCT images when acquiring the scan for the purpose of implant/surgical planning [85,86]. The most common IFs encompass concha bullosa, mucosal thickening, polyps, altered sinus dimensions, and sinus opacification. Some IFs may also be suggestive of benign or malignant neoplastic processes. Hence, it is important for the dental practitioner to be aware of these findings on CBCT images, which might allow a more appropriate selection of a treatment plan as patients with IFs might be redisposed to a higher risk of postoperative complications from SFE and implant placement. Although a smaller FOV CBCT scan results in less radiation, the risk of missing IFs still exists. Hence, it is recommended to acquire a scan with an optimal FOV depending on the clinical indications and risk–benefit analysis. To reach a more definitive conclusion, more research is also needed to examine how different FOVs affect the incidence of IFs.

3. Digital Workflow for SFE Procedures

In recent years, digital technologies and workflows have been introduced in the majority of dental medicine fields, including restorative dentistry, orthodontics, dental implantology, and maxillofacial reconstructive surgery [87]. Digital treatment planning workflow refers to the incorporation of computer-controlled components and dental technologies for assisting a clinician with the planning process. This digitization of workflows in clinical dentistry has overcome the limitations associated with traditional methods by offering improved precision of dental procedures, time-efficiency, and a higher standard of patient care [88–90].

3.1. Virtual Modelling

Generally, CBCT images are saved in a Digital Imaging and Communications in Medicine (DICOM) format, which is then transferred to 3D software programs for further processing to plan the procedure. The most essential step in SFE planning workflows is segmentation, a process by which the region of interest is extracted from 3D images for generating 3D virtual models. These models are then used for fabricating guides or pre-surgically assessing the amount of required (bone) graft (Figure 1).

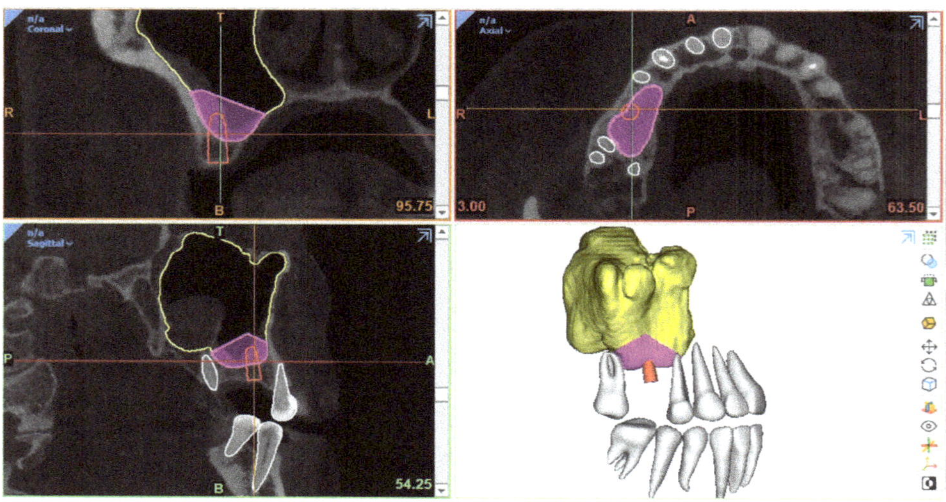

Figure 1. Example of graft volume estimation in Mimics (version 23.0, Materialise N.V., Leuven, Belgium) following automated sinus and teeth segmentation (creator.relu.eu, Relu, BV, Version March 2023).

Traditionally, manual sinus segmentation, referred to as slice-by-slice delineation on 2D CBCT planes, performed by an expert is considered the gold standard. However, it is prone to certain limitations, such as labor-intensiveness, increased time consumption, and observer variability [91,92]. Based on the aforementioned limitations, semi-automated segmentation via thresholding-based approaches has been widely adopted for the segmentation of CBCT images to improve the efficiency of planning workflows [93,94]. Nevertheless, the final segmentation lacks optimal delineation due to the presence of different structural densities, and manual post-processing is often required. Recently, artificial intelligence (AI) in the form of deep learning has been employed for automated segmentation to overcome the limitations associated with both manual and semi-automated segmentation approaches. In deep learning, convolutional neural networks (CNNs) have demonstrated excellent performance with the employment of multi-layer neural computational connections for sinus segmentation on CBCT images [95–97]. The application of such deep learning-based approaches might enhance the quality and predictability of presurgical graft planning, enable a more precise treatment planning process and volumetric quantification of sinus/graft changes, and may further improve the standard of care. Yet, a lack of evidence exists related to the application of AI in the SFE treatment planning workflows.

3.2. *Surgical Guidance*

In SFE procedures, CBCT-based guidance has played a vital role in improving the precision of the surgical procedure with a reduction in complications. The guidance can be static or dynamic in nature. The procedures performed via these guides are referred to as "guided sinus lift [98]" or "guided bone grafting [99]".

3.2.1. Static Surgical Guides

Static guides are designed via 3D planning software programs following the integration of intraoral scanned images with CBCT datasets and later fabricated using 3D printers. Such surgical templates act as a support aid and offer the advantages of time-efficiency, better working ergonomics, less operator stress, and greater predictability of the procedure [98,100,101]. Moreover, this procedure can also be combined with concurrent implant placement planning.

In 2008, Manderales and Rosenfeld [99] pioneered computer-guided SFE. They proposed using CAD/CAM surgical cutting guides for exact lateral wall outlining to considerably improve the quality and outcomes of the SFE procedure. Cecchetti et al. [98] have recently introduced virtual planning of surgical guides for lateral wall sinus elevation, concluding that the surgical template should be seen as a support aid to minimize risk and complications of the surgical procedures, especially in "difficult" cases.

Following the same concept, Osman et al. [102] and Strbac et al. [101] performed computer-guided SFE through a lateral window approach in addition to simultaneous implant placement. They found that applying static guides resulted in better and more consistent results. Similarly, Pistilli et al. [100] also concluded that such a digital approach is highly efficient in the mid-term (follow-up of 10 years) to implant rehabilitation of severely resorbed maxilla simultaneously with sinus lift.

Considering transrectal sinus augmentation, Pozzi et al. [103] and An et al. [104] combined static guide-based flapless maxillary crestal sinus augmentation with an immediate nonfunctional loading of dental implants, reporting a 98.53% and 100% survival rate at 3 years and 37 months, respectively.

Another type of surgical guidance is dynamic navigation, which is based on computer-guided surgery planning. Here, a physical surgical guide is unnecessary [105].

3.2.2. Dynamic Surgical Guides

A dynamic navigation system combined with CBCT imaging has been proposed for improving the intraoperative precision of implant placement, where a static surgical guide is not required and the operator can place the implants with real-time navigation [106]. With regard to SFE, limited evidence exists related to the application of navigation-based approaches. Recently, dynamic navigation has been used for posterior maxilla implant surgery via transcrestal SFE using piezoelectric devices [107]. The proposed technique offered high precision with excellent clinical outcome. However, it is recommended to perform further clinical studies to assess the effectiveness of dynamic navigation for performing SFE.

Considering the intraoperative use of CBCT imaging, Blake et al. [108] performed one case trial of using a C-arm-based CBCT scanner during sinus augmentation surgery under general anesthesia with iliac crest grafting. The images were taken prior to wound closure to immediately verify the surgery result. However, there is no solid evidence regarding such procedures for surgeries performed under local anesthesia.

4. Use of CBCT for Monitoring and Follow-Up after SFE

Post-surgical radiographic examination is vital [19,49,109–121] for the evaluation of bony integration of the inserted graft, follow-up of its long term stability, and also assessment of implant success and/or osteointegration after sinus lift procedures.

Ideally, imaging guidelines for the follow-up of sinus augmentation with or without immediate implant placement should follow the same regulations as those for post-surgical implant placement. Based on the AAOMR recommendations [55] and the guidelines for the use of diagnostic imaging in implant dentistry published by the E.A.O. [56], intraoral periapical radiography should be performed for the postoperative assessment of implants in the absence of clinical signs or symptoms. Panoramic radiographs may be indicated for more extensive implant therapy cases.

Meanwhile, CBCT [109,112,115] has become the standard imaging technique for 3D visualization and improved assessment prior to implant placement in the case of staged sinus augmentation. CBCT imaging can help to assess bone healing by visualizing how the material has integrated with the surrounding bone as well as if any signs of early resorption exist. It is beneficial in providing information about the volume, extent, and density of the augmented region [56] and can also be used to monitor any complications, which are not visible to the naked eye, such as mucosal changes, infection, and/or inflammation.

Furthermore, bone graft materials undergo remodeling over time at varying rates depending on the material used (resorbable versus non-resorbable) [122], and positive pressure formed inside the sinus during respiration also accelerates graft resorption [123]. Certainly, this remodeling could have a significant impact on the success of SFE outcome and the respective implant treatment. Thereby, CBCT can aid in the quantification of the resorption rate of different grafting materials [124–126] and also to monitor sinus changes at follow-up stages by comparing pre-surgical and/or post-surgical scans acquired at different time points. Usually, the Schneiderian membrane exhibits significant post-surgical edema, which increases the mucosal thickness visible. In addition, the edema might cause ostium obstruction with the possibility of impaired drainage capacity of sinus mucus. The reduction in the patency and obstruction of the ostium and infundibulum can lead to an inflammatory reaction and/or infectious processes of the sinus cavity, causing acute or chronic sinusitis [127]. Hence, CBCT imaging could act as a useful follow-up assessment tool to measure the thickness of the membrane and monitor mucosal changes in an attempt to avoid both early and delayed postoperative complications [128]. Additionally, following up the mucosal thickness changes could help to study the possible effects of different graft materials on sinus mucosa for research purposes [129].

It should be kept in mind that the use of CBCT should not be opted for regular follow-up assessment of normal SFE procedures without any evident or suspected complications to avoid exposure to unnecessary radiation doses. Postoperative CBCT could be indicated in cases with complications and contraindicated in patients where no direct benefit is to be expected. In instances of no clinical signs or symptoms of treatment failure or complications, periapical or panoramic images could be considered more than enough for postoperative follow-up. Moreover, CBCT imaging should also be justifiable for ethically approved clinical research projects, which might improve the standard of patient care. However, optimized strategies still need to be developed for SFE follow-up assessment, allowing good image quality and accurate 3D modeling with low-dose scanning protocols.

5. Recommendations and Future Developments

Maxillary sinus floor elevation is nowadays considered a safe and effective surgical technique to allow prosthetic restoration supported by implants in the atrophic posterior region of the maxilla. CBCT imaging has significantly improved the accuracy and efficiency of performing SFE procedures. It has become an imaging modality of choice for diagnostics due to its potential for detecting challenging anatomical and/or pathological entities, which would probably remain undetected with 2D imaging. However, one should consider that in a private practice, it is difficult and time consuming for a dentist to identify all CBCT-based diagnostic parameters, which might negatively impact the decision-making process. Hence, future studies should attempt to integrate artificial intelligence-based solutions using CBCT images for automating and standardizing the diagnostic and decision-making process for performing SFE procedure.

In relation to treatment planning, automated AI-based CBCT image segmentation has already been implemented for the production of virtual models of maxillary sinuses and jawbone. However, still no evidence exists related to the integration of AI networks in the digital treatment planning workflows of SFE. Hence, future studies should also focus on investigating the accuracy and efficiency of these networks and models in treatment planning workflows. Furthermore, they should also investigate the combination of quantitative extracted features following image segmentation with biological, clinical, and demographic patient characteristics, which is referred to as "radiomics" [130]. Such a combination could be a step forward toward personalized dental medicine, enabling the best possible treatment for each patient [131,132].

As for follow-up assessments, it is recommended to perform studies comparing the 3D resorption rate associated with different surgical techniques and grafting materials and also assess the morphological changes of the sinus. Even for the post-surgical assessment of the sinus and grafted region, the application of AI allowing automated virtual modeling could be beneficial in an attempt to further improve the surgical outcomes and better understand the associated complications. As for the justification of CBCT imaging, there is a need for future research to establish an optimized low-dose CBCT protocol for SFE diagnostics, 3D planning, and follow-up assessment, which does not impair the image quality depending on the task at hand.

Funding: This research received no external funding.

Institutional Review Board Statement: Not applicable.

Informed Consent Statement: Not applicable.

Data Availability Statement: Data sharing is not applicable to this article.

Conflicts of Interest: The authors declare no conflict of interest.

References

1. Chen, S.T.; Darby, I. Alveolar ridge preservation and early implant placement at maxillary central incisor sites: A prospective case series study. *Clin. Oral Implant. Res.* **2020**, *31*, 803–813. [CrossRef] [PubMed]
2. Hansson, S.; Halldin, A. Alveolar ridge resorption after tooth extraction: A consequence of a fundamental principle of bone physiology. *J. Dent. Biomech.* **2012**, *3*, 1758736012456543. [CrossRef] [PubMed]
3. Farmer, M.; Darby, I. Ridge dimensional changes following single-tooth extraction in the aesthetic zone. *Clin. Oral Implant. Res.* **2014**, *25*, 272–277. [CrossRef] [PubMed]
4. Jemt, T.; Lekholm, U. Implant treatment in edentulous maxillae: A 5-year follow-up report on patients with different degrees of jaw resorption. *Int. J. Oral Maxillofac. Implant.* **1995**, *10*, 303–311.
5. Bathla, S.C.; Fry, R.R.; Majumdar, K. Maxillary sinus augmentation. *J. Indian Soc. Periodontol.* **2018**, *22*, 468–473. [CrossRef] [PubMed]
6. Bornstein, M.M.; Chappuis, V.; Von Arx, T.; Buser, D. Performance of dental implants after staged sinus floor elevation procedures: 5-year results of a prospective study in partially edentulous patients. *Clin. Oral Implant. Res.* **2008**, *19*, 1034–1043. [CrossRef]
7. Del Fabbro, M.; Wallace, S.S.; Testori, T. Long-term implant survival in the grafted maxillary sinus: A systematic review. *Int. J. Periodontics Restor. Dent.* **2013**, *33*, 773–783. [CrossRef]
8. Esposito, M.; Felice, P.; Worthington, H.V. Interventions for replacing missing teeth: Augmentation procedures of the maxillary sinus. *Cochrane Database Syst. Rev.* **2014**, Cd008397. [CrossRef]
9. Starch-Jensen, T.; Jensen, J.D. Maxillary Sinus Floor Augmentation: A Review of Selected Treatment Modalities. *J. Oral Maxillofac. Res.* **2017**, *8*, e3. [CrossRef]
10. Boyne, P.J.; James, R.A. Grafting of the maxillary sinus floor with autogenous marrow and bone. *J. Oral Surg.* **1980**, *38*, 613–616.

11. Caudry, S.; Landzberg, M. Lateral window sinus elevation technique: Managing challenges and complications. *J. Can. Dent. Assoc.* **2013**, *79*, d101. [PubMed]
12. Tatum, H., Jr. Maxillary and sinus implant reconstructions. *Dent. Clin. N. Am.* **1986**, *30*, 207–229. [CrossRef] [PubMed]
13. Summers, R.B. A new concept in maxillary implant surgery: The osteotome technique. *Compendium* **1994**, *15*, 152, 154-6, 158 passim; quiz 162.
14. Temmerman, A.; Van Dessel, J.; Cortellini, S.; Jacobs, R.; Teughels, W.; Quirynen, M. Volumetric changes of grafted volumes and the Schneiderian membrane after transcrestal and lateral sinus floor elevation procedures: A clinical, pilot study. *J. Clin. Periodontol.* **2017**, *44*, 660–671. [CrossRef]
15. Wang, H.L.; Katranji, A. ABC sinus augmentation classification. *Int. J. Periodontics Restor. Dent.* **2008**, *28*, 383–389.
16. Mohan, N.; Wolf, J.; Dym, H. Maxillary sinus augmentation. *Dent. Clin. N. Am.* **2015**, *59*, 375–388. [CrossRef]
17. Zhao, R.; Yang, R.; Cooper, P.R.; Khurshid, Z.; Shavandi, A.; Ratnayake, J. Bone Grafts and Substitutes in Dentistry: A Review of Current Trends and Developments. *Molecules* **2021**, *26*, 3007. [CrossRef]
18. Johansson, L.A.; Isaksson, S.; Lindh, C.; Becktor, J.P.; Sennerby, L. Maxillary sinus floor augmentation and simultaneous implant placement using locally harvested autogenous bone chips and bone debris: A prospective clinical study. *J. Oral Maxillofac. Surg.* **2010**, *68*, 837–844. [CrossRef]
19. Klijn, R.J.; Meijer, G.J.; Bronkhorst, E.M.; Jansen, J.A. A meta-analysis of histomorphometric results and graft healing time of various biomaterials compared to autologous bone used as sinus floor augmentation material in humans. *Tissue Eng. Part B Rev.* **2010**, *16*, 493–507. [CrossRef] [PubMed]
20. Nkenke, E.; Stelzle, F. Clinical outcomes of sinus floor augmentation for implant placement using autogenous bone or bone substitutes: A systematic review. *Clin. Oral Implant. Res.* **2009**, *20* (Suppl. S4), 124–133. [CrossRef]
21. Schmitt, C.M.; Doering, H.; Schmidt, T.; Lutz, R.; Neukam, F.W.; Schlegel, K.A. Histological results after maxillary sinus augmentation with Straumann®BoneCeramic, Bio-Oss®, Puros®, and autologous bone. A randomized controlled clinical trial. *Clin. Oral Implant. Res.* **2013**, *24*, 576–585. [CrossRef] [PubMed]
22. Maiorana, C.; Ferrario, S.; Poli, P.P.; Manfredini, M. Autogenous Chin Block Grafts in the Aesthetic Zone: A 20-Year Follow-Up Case Report. *Case Rep. Dent.* **2020**, *2020*, 6525797. [CrossRef]
23. Reininger, D.; Cobo-Vázquez, C.; Rosenberg, B.; López-Quiles, J. Alternative intraoral donor sites to the chin and mandibular body-ramus. *J. Clin. Exp. Dent.* **2017**, *9*, e1474–e1481. [CrossRef] [PubMed]
24. Sakkas, A.; Wilde, F.; Heufelder, M.; Winter, K.; Schramm, A. Autogenous bone grafts in oral implantology—Is it still a "gold standard"? A consecutive review of 279 patients with 456 clinical procedures. *Int. J. Implant. Dent.* **2017**, *3*, 23. [CrossRef]
25. Titsinides, S.; Agrogiannis, G.; Karatzas, T. Bone grafting materials in dentoalveolar reconstruction: A comprehensive review. *Jpn. Dent. Sci. Rev.* **2019**, *55*, 26–32. [CrossRef]
26. Wortmann, D.E.; Klein-Nulend, J.; van Ruijven, L.J.; Schortinghuis, J.; Vissink, A.; Raghoebar, G.M. Incorporation of anterior iliac crest or calvarial bone grafts in reconstructed atrophied maxillae: A randomized clinical trial with histomorphometric and micro-CT analyses. *Clin. Implant. Dent. Relat. Res.* **2021**, *23*, 492–502. [CrossRef]
27. Annibali, S.; Cristalli, M.P.; La Monaca, G.; Bignozzi, I.; Scarano, A.; Corrado, R.; Muzio, L.L. Human maxillary sinuses augmented with mineralized, solvent-dehydrated bone allograft: A longitudinal case series. *Implant. Dent.* **2011**, *20*, 445–454. [CrossRef] [PubMed]
28. Bavetta, G. The use of human allogenic graft (HBA) for maxillary bone regeneration: Review of literature and case reports. *Curr. Pharm. Des.* **2012**, *18*, 5559–5568. [CrossRef]
29. Irinakis, T. Efficacy of injectable demineralized bone matrix as graft material during sinus elevation surgery with simultaneous implant placement in the posterior maxilla: Clinical evaluation of 49 sinuses. *J. Oral Maxillofac. Surg.* **2011**, *69*, 134–141. [CrossRef]
30. Chaushu, L.; Silva, E.R.; Balan, V.F.; Chaushu, G.; Xavier, S.P. Sinus augmentation-autograft vs. fresh frozen allograft: Bone density dynamics and implant stability. *J. Stomatol. Oral Maxillofac. Surg.* **2021**, *122*, 467–471. [CrossRef]
31. Roberts, T.T.; Rosenbaum, A.J. Bone grafts, bone substitutes and orthobiologics. *Organogenesis* **2012**, *8*, 114–124. [CrossRef]
32. Özkan, Y.; Akoğlu, B.; Kulak-Özkan, Y. Maxillary sinus floor augmentation using bovine bone grafts with simultaneous implant placement: A 5-year prospective follow-up study. *Implant. Dent.* **2011**, *20*, 455–459. [CrossRef]
33. Scarano, A.; Piattelli, A.; Perrotti, V.; Manzon, L.; Iezzi, G. Maxillary sinus augmentation in humans using cortical porcine bone: A histological and histomorphometrical evaluation after 4 and 6 months. *Clin. Implant. Dent. Relat. Res.* **2011**, *13*, 13–18. [CrossRef]
34. Sivolella, S.; Bressan, E.; Gnocco, E.; Berengo, M.; Favero, G.A. Maxillary sinus augmentation with bovine bone and simultaneous dental implant placement in conditions of severe alveolar atrophy: A retrospective analysis of a consecutively treated case series. *Quintessence Int.* **2011**, *42*, 851–862. [PubMed]
35. Temmerman, A.; Cortellini, S.; Van Dessel, J.; De Greef, A.; Jacobs, R.; Dhondt, R.; Teughels, W.; Quirynen, M. Bovine-derived xenograft in combination with autogenous bone chips versus xenograft alone for the augmentation of bony dehiscences around oral implants: A randomized, controlled, split-mouth clinical trial. *J. Clin. Periodontol.* **2020**, *47*, 110–119. [CrossRef] [PubMed]
36. Testori, T.; Iezzi, G.; Manzon, L.; Fratto, G.; Piattelli, A.; Weinstein, R.L. High temperature-treated bovine porous hydroxyapatite in sinus augmentation procedures: A case report. *Int. J. Periodontics Restor. Dent.* **2012**, *32*, 295–301.
37. Kuchler, U.; Dos Santos, G.M.; Heimel, P.; Stähli, A.; Strauss, F.J.; Tangl, S.; Gruber, R. DBBM shows no signs of resorption under inflammatory conditions. An experimental study in the mouse calvaria. *Clin. Oral Implant. Res.* **2020**, *31*, 10–17. [CrossRef]

38. Kuchler, U.; Heimel, P.; Stähli, A.; Strauss, F.J.; Luza, B.; Gruber, R. Impact of DBBM Fragments on the Porosity of the Calvarial Bone: A Pilot Study on Mice. *Materials* **2020**, *13*, 4748. [CrossRef]
39. Sheikh, Z.; Hamdan, N.; Abdallah, M.-N.; Glogauer, M.; Grynpas, M. Natural and synthetic bone replacement graft materials for dental and maxillofacial applications. In *Advanced Dental Biomaterials*; Khurshid, Z., Najeeb, S., Zafar, M.S., Sefat, F., Eds.; Woodhead Publishing: Sawston, UK, 2019; pp. 347–376.
40. Kolk, A.; Handschel, J.; Drescher, W.; Rothamel, D.; Kloss, F.; Blessmann, M.; Heiland, M.; Wolff, K.-D.; Smeets, R. Current trends and future perspectives of bone substitute materials–from space holders to innovative biomaterials. *J. Cranio-Maxillofac. Surg.* **2012**, *40*, 706–718. [CrossRef]
41. Wang, W.; Yeung, K.W.K. Bone grafts and biomaterials substitutes for bone defect repair: A review. *Bioact. Mater.* **2017**, *2*, 224–247. [CrossRef]
42. Temmerman, A.; Hertelé, S.; Teughels, W.; Dekeyser, C.; Jacobs, R.; Quirynen, M. Are panoramic images reliable in planning sinus augmentation procedures? *Clin. Oral Implant. Res.* **2011**, *22*, 189–194. [CrossRef] [PubMed]
43. Bornstein, M.M.; Horner, K.; Jacobs, R. Use of cone beam computed tomography in implant dentistry: Current concepts, indications and limitations for clinical practice and research. *Periodontology 2000* **2017**, *73*, 51–72. [CrossRef]
44. Bornstein, M.M.; Scarfe, W.C.; Vaughn, V.M.; Jacobs, R. Cone beam computed tomography in implant dentistry: A systematic review focusing on guidelines, indications, and radiation dose risks. *Int. J. Oral Maxillofac. Implant.* **2014**, *29*, 55–77. [CrossRef]
45. Jacobs, R.; Salmon, B.; Codari, M.; Hassan, B.; Bornstein, M.M. Cone beam computed tomography in implant dentistry: Recommendations for clinical use. *BMC Oral Health* **2018**, *18*, 88. [CrossRef]
46. Reddy, M.S.; Mayfield-Donahoo, T.; Vanderven, F.J.; Jeffcoat, M.K. A comparison of the diagnostic advantages of panoramic radiography and computed tomography scanning for placement of root form dental implants. *Clin. Oral Implant. Res.* **1994**, *5*, 229–238. [CrossRef] [PubMed]
47. Arias-Irimia, Ó.; Barona Dorado, C.; Gómez Moreno, G.; Brinkmann, J.C.; Martínez-González, J.M. Pre-operative measurement of the volume of bone graft in sinus lifts using CompuDent. *Clin. Oral Implant. Res.* **2012**, *23*, 1070–1074. [CrossRef] [PubMed]
48. Buyukkurt, M.C.; Tozoglu, S.; Yavuz, M.S.; Aras, M.H. Simulation of sinus floor augmentation with symphysis bone graft using three-dimensional computerized tomography. *Int. J. Oral Maxillofac. Surg.* **2010**, *39*, 788–792. [CrossRef]
49. Krennmair, G.; Krainhöfner, M.; Maier, H.; Weinländer, M.; Piehslinger, E. Computerized tomography-assisted calculation of sinus augmentation volume. *Int. J. Oral Maxillofac. Implant.* **2006**, *21*, 907–913.
50. Uchida, Y.; Goto, M.; Katsuki, T.; Soejima, Y. Measurement of maxillary sinus volume using computerized tomographic images. *Int. J. Oral Maxillofac. Implant.* **1998**, *13*, 811–818.
51. Scarfe, W.C.; Farman, A.G. What is cone-beam CT and how does it work? *Dent. Clin. N. Am.* **2008**, *52*, 707–730. [CrossRef]
52. Scarfe, W.C.; Farman, A.G.; Sukovic, P. Clinical applications of cone-beam computed tomography in dental practice. *J. Can. Dent. Assoc.* **2006**, *72*, 75–80. [PubMed]
53. White, S.C.; Pharoah, M.J. *White and Pharoah's Oral Radiology: Principles and Interpretation*; Elsevier Health Sciences: Amsterdam, The Netherlands, 2018; pp. 418–444.
54. Pauwels, R.; Jacobs, R.; Singer, S.R.; Mupparapu, M. CBCT-based bone quality assessment: Are Hounsfield units applicable? *Dentomaxillofacial Radiol.* **2015**, *44*, 20140238. [CrossRef]
55. Tyndall, D.A.; Price, J.B.; Tetradis, S.; Ganz, S.D.; Hildebolt, C.; Scarfe, W.C. Position statement of the American Academy of Oral and Maxillofacial Radiology on selection criteria for the use of radiology in dental implantology with emphasis on cone beam computed tomography. *Oral Surg. Oral Med. Oral Pathol. Oral Radiol.* **2012**, *113*, 817–826. [CrossRef]
56. Harris, D.; Horner, K.; Gröndahl, K.; Jacobs, R.; Helmrot, E.; Benic, G.I.; Bornstein, M.M.; Dawood, A.; Quirynen, M.E.A.O. guidelines for the use of diagnostic imaging in implant dentistry 2011. A consensus workshop organized by the European Association for Osseointegration at the Medical University of Warsaw. *Clin. Oral Implant. Res.* **2012**, *23*, 1243–1253. [CrossRef] [PubMed]
57. Oenning, A.C.; Jacobs, R.; Pauwels, R.; Stratis, A.; Hedesiu, M.; Salmon, B. Cone-beam CT in paediatric dentistry: DIMITRA project position statement. *Pediatr. Radiol.* **2018**, *48*, 308–316. [CrossRef]
58. Oenning, A.C.; Jacobs, R.; Salmon, B. ALADAIP, beyond ALARA and towards personalized optimization for paediatric cone-beam CT. *Int. J. Paediatr. Dent.* **2021**, *31*, 676–678. [CrossRef]
59. Carmeli, G.; Artzi, Z.; Kozlovsky, A.; Segev, Y.; Landsberg, R. Antral computerized tomography pre-operative evaluation: Relationship between mucosal thickening and maxillary sinus function. *Clin. Oral Implant. Res.* **2011**, *22*, 78–82. [CrossRef] [PubMed]
60. Janner, S.F.; Caversaccio, M.D.; Dubach, P.; Sendi, P.; Buser, D.; Bornstein, M.M. Characteristics and dimensions of the Schneiderian membrane: A radiographic analysis using cone beam computed tomography in patients referred for dental implant surgery in the posterior maxilla. *Clin. Oral Implant. Res.* **2011**, *22*, 1446–1453. [CrossRef]
61. Pignataro, L.; Mantovani, M.; Torretta, S.; Felisati, G.; Sambataro, G. ENT assessment in the integrated management of candidate for (maxillary) sinus lift. *Acta Otorhinolaryngol. Ital.* **2008**, *28*, 110–119.
62. Ribeiro-Rotta, R.F.; Lindh, C.; Pereira, A.C.; Rohlin, M. Ambiguity in bone tissue characteristics as presented in studies on dental implant planning and placement: A systematic review. *Clin. Oral Implant. Res.* **2011**, *22*, 789–801. [CrossRef]
63. Pauwels, R.; Araki, K.; Siewerdsen, J.H.; Thongvigitmanee, S.S. Technical aspects of dental CBCT: State of the art. *Dentomaxillofacial Radiol.* **2015**, *44*, 20140224. [CrossRef]

64. Loubele, M.; Bogaerts, R.; Van Dijck, E.; Pauwels, R.; Vanheusden, S.; Suetens, P.; Marchal, G.; Sanderink, G.; Jacobs, R. Comparison between effective radiation dose of CBCT and MSCT scanners for dentomaxillofacial applications. *Eur. J. Radiol.* **2009**, *71*, 461–468. [CrossRef]
65. Rahpeyma, A.; Khajehahmadi, S. Open Sinus Lift Surgery and the Importance of Preoperative Cone-Beam Computed Tomography Scan: A Review. *J. Int. Oral Health* **2015**, *7*, 127–133.
66. Ducommun, J.; Bornstein, M.M.; Wong, M.C.M.; von Arx, T. Distances of root apices to adjacent anatomical structures in the anterior maxilla: An analysis using cone beam computed tomography. *Clin. Oral Investig.* **2019**, *23*, 2253–2263. [CrossRef] [PubMed]
67. Kahnberg, K.-E.; Wallström, M.; Rasmusson, L. Local sinus lift for single-tooth implant. I. clinical and radiographic follow-up. *Clin. Implant. Dent. Relat. Res.* **2011**, *13*, 231–237. [CrossRef]
68. Testori, T.; Weinstein, T.; Taschieri, S.; Wallace, S.S. Risk factors in lateral window sinus elevation surgery. *Periodontology 2000* **2019**, *81*, 91–123. [CrossRef]
69. Janner, S.F.M.; Dubach, P.; Suter, V.G.A.; Caversaccio, M.D.; Buser, D.; Bornstein, M.M. Sinus floor elevation or referral for further diagnosis and therapy: A comparison of maxillary sinus assessment by ENT specialists and dentists using cone beam computed tomography. *Clin. Oral Implant. Res.* **2020**, *31*, 463–475. [CrossRef]
70. Becker, S.T.; Terheyden, H.; Steinriede, A.; Behrens, E.; Springer, I.; Wiltfang, J. Prospective observation of 41 perforations of the Schneiderian membrane during sinus floor elevation. *Clin. Oral Implant. Res.* **2008**, *19*, 1285–1289. [CrossRef]
71. Monje, A.; Diaz, K.T.; Aranda, L.; Insua, A.; Garcia-Nogales, A.; Wang, H.-L. Schneiderian Membrane Thickness and Clinical Implications for Sinus Augmentation: A Systematic Review and Meta-Regression Analyses. *J. Periodontol.* **2016**, *87*, 888–899. [CrossRef] [PubMed]
72. Tavelli, L.; Borgonovo, A.E.; Re, D.; Maiorana, C. Sinus presurgical evaluation: A literature review and a new classification proposal. *Minerva Stomatol.* **2017**, *66*, 115–131. [CrossRef] [PubMed]
73. Shanbhag, S.; Karnik, P.; Shirke, P.; Shanbhag, V. Cone-beam computed tomographic analysis of sinus membrane thickness, ostium patency, and residual ridge heights in the posterior maxilla: Implications for sinus floor elevation. *Clin. Oral Implant. Res.* **2013**, *25*, 755–760. [CrossRef] [PubMed]
74. Bornstein, M.M.; Seiffert, C.; Maestre-Ferrín, L.; Fodich, I.; Jacobs, R.; Buser, D.; Von Arx, T. An Analysis of Frequency, Morphology, and Locations of Maxillary Sinus Septa Using Cone Beam Computed Tomography. *Int. J. Oral Maxillofac. Implant.* **2016**, *31*, 280–287. [CrossRef]
75. Schriber, M.; Von Arx, T.; Sendi, P.; Jacobs, R.; Suter, V.G.; Bornstein, M.M. Evaluating Maxillary Sinus Septa Using Cone Beam Computed Tomography: Is There a Difference in Frequency and Type Between the Dentate and Edentulous Posterior Maxilla? *Int. J. Oral Maxillofac. Implant.* **2017**, *32*, 1324–1332. [CrossRef]
76. Neugebauer, J.; Ritter, L.; Mischkowski, R.A.; Dreiseidler, T.; Scherer, P.; Ketterle, M.; Rothamel, D.; Zöller, J.E. Evaluation of maxillary sinus anatomy by cone-beam CT prior to sinus floor elevation. *Int. J. Oral Maxillofac. Implant.* **2010**, *25*, 258–265.
77. Zijderveld, S.A.; van den Bergh, J.P.; Schulten, E.A.; ten Bruggenkate, C.M. Anatomical and surgical findings and complications in 100 consecutive maxillary sinus floor elevation procedures. *J. Oral Maxillofac. Surg.* **2008**, *66*, 1426–1438. [CrossRef]
78. Yeung, A.W.K.; Colsoul, N.; Montalvao, C.; Hung, K.; Jacobs, R.; Bornstein, M.M. Visibility, location, and morphology of the primary maxillary sinus ostium and presence of accessory ostia: A retrospective analysis using cone beam computed tomography (CBCT). *Clin. Oral Investig.* **2019**, *23*, 3977–3986. [CrossRef]
79. Chan, H.-L.; Suarez, F.; Monje, A.; Benavides, E.; Wang, H.-L. Evaluation of maxillary sinus width on cone-beam computed tomography for sinus augmentation and new sinus classification based on sinus width. *Clin. Oral Implant. Res.* **2012**, *25*, 647–652. [CrossRef] [PubMed]
80. Lim, E.L.; Ngeow, W.C.; Lim, D. The implications of different lateral wall thicknesses on surgical access to the maxillary sinus. *Braz. Oral Res.* **2017**, *31*, e97. [CrossRef] [PubMed]
81. Varela-Centelles, P.; Loira, M.; González-Mosquera, A.; Romero-Mendez, A.; Seoane, J.; García-Pola, M.J.; Seoane-Romero, J.M. Study of factors influencing preoperative detection of alveolar antral artery by CBCT in sinus floor elevation. *Sci. Rep.* **2020**, *10*, 10820. [CrossRef] [PubMed]
82. Greenstein, G.; Cavallaro, J.; Tarnow, D. Practical application of anatomy for the dental implant surgeon. *J. Periodontol.* **2008**, *79*, 1833–1846. [CrossRef]
83. Jacobs, R.; Scarfe, W.C. Dental Implants. In *Maxillofacial Cone Beam Computed Tomography: Principles, Techniques and Clinical Applications*; Scarfe, W.C., Angelopoulos, C., Eds.; Springer International Publishing: Cham, Switzerland, 2018; pp. 745–830.
84. Abdel-Wahed, N.A.; Bahammam, M.A. Cone Beam CT-Based Preoperative Volumetric Estimation of Bone Graft Required for Lateral Window Sinus Augmentation, Compared with Intraoperative Findings: A Pilot Study. *Open Dent. J.* **2018**, *12*, 820–826. [CrossRef]
85. Binshabaib, M.; Alharthi, S.; Alkraida, R.; Aljared, S.; Alshami, A.; Mansour, S. Incidental findings in maxillary sinus area on cone-beam-computed-tomographic-scans: A retrospective study with emphasis on gender and ethnicity. *Saudi Dent. J.* **2021**, *33*, 184–187. [CrossRef]
86. Pazera, P.; Bornstein, M.M.; Pazera, A.; Sendi, P.; Katsaros, C. Incidental maxillary sinus findings in orthodontic patients: A radiographic analysis using cone-beam computed tomography (CBCT). *Orthod. Craniofacial Res.* **2011**, *14*, 17–24. [CrossRef] [PubMed]

87. Vandenberghe, B. The digital patient–Imaging science in dentistry. *J. Dent.* **2018**, *74* (Suppl. S1), S21–S26. [CrossRef]
88. Lin, Y.-M. Digitalisation in Dentistry: Development and Practices. In *The Digitization of Business in China: Exploring the Transformation from Manufacturing to a Digital Service Hub*; Kim, Y.-C., Chen, P.-C., Eds.; Springer International Publishing: Cham, Switzerland, 2018; pp. 199–217.
89. Shujaat, S.; Bornstein, M.M.; Price, J.B.; Jacobs, R. Integration of imaging modalities in digital dental workflows-possibilities, limitations, and potential future developments. *Dentomaxillofacial Radiol.* **2021**, *50*, 20210268. [CrossRef] [PubMed]
90. Shujaat, S.; Riaz, M.; Jacobs, R. Synergy between artificial intelligence and precision medicine for computer-assisted oral and maxillofacial surgical planning. *Clin. Oral Investig.* **2023**, *27*, 897–906. [CrossRef] [PubMed]
91. Heye, T.; Merkle, E.M.; Reiner, C.S.; Davenport, M.S.; Horvath, J.J.; Feuerlein, S.; Breault, S.R.; Gall, P.; Bashir, M.R.; Dale, B.M.; et al. Reproducibility of dynamic contrast-enhanced MR imaging. Part II. Comparison of intra- and interobserver variability with manual region of interest placement versus semiautomatic lesion segmentation and histogram analysis. *Radiology* **2013**, *266*, 812–821. [CrossRef] [PubMed]
92. Parmar, C.; Velazquez, E.R.; Leijenaar, R.; Jermoumi, M.; Carvalho, S.; Mak, R.H.; Mitra, S.; Shankar, B.U.; Kikinis, R.; Haibe-Kains, B.; et al. Robust Radiomics feature quantification using semiautomatic volumetric segmentation. *PLoS ONE* **2014**, *9*, e102107. [CrossRef]
93. Renard, F.; Guedria, S.; De Palma, N.; Vuillerme, N. Variability and reproducibility in deep learning for medical image segmentation. *Sci. Rep.* **2020**, *10*, 13724. [CrossRef]
94. Withey, D.; Koles, Z. Medical Image Segmentation: Methods and Software. In Proceedings of the 2007 Joint Meeting of the 6th International Symposium on Noninvasive Functional Source Imaging of the Brain and Heart and the International Conference on Functional Biomedical Imaging, Hangzhou, China, 12–14 October 2007; pp. 140–143. [CrossRef]
95. Choi, H.; Jeon, K.J.; Kim, Y.H.; Ha, E.-G.; Lee, C.; Han, S.-S. Deep learning-based fully automatic segmentation of the maxillary sinus on cone-beam computed tomographic images. *Sci. Rep.* **2022**, *12*, 14009. [CrossRef] [PubMed]
96. Hung, K.F.; Ai, Q.Y.H.; King, A.D.; Bornstein, M.M.; Wong, L.M.; Leung, Y.Y. Automatic detection and segmentation of morphological changes of the maxillary sinus mucosa on cone-beam computed tomography images using a three-dimensional convolutional neural network. *Clin. Oral Investig.* **2022**, *26*, 3987–3998. [CrossRef] [PubMed]
97. Jung, S.-K.; Lim, H.-K.; Lee, S.; Cho, Y.; Song, I.-S. Deep Active Learning for Automatic Segmentation of Maxillary Sinus Lesions Using a Convolutional Neural Network. *Diagnostics* **2021**, *11*, 688. [CrossRef]
98. Cecchetti, F.; Spuntarelli, M.; Mazza, D.; Di Girolamo, M.; Baggi, L. Guided sinus lift: Virtual planning of surgical templates for lateral access. *J. Biol. Regul. Homeost. Agents* **2021**, *35*, 139–145. [CrossRef] [PubMed]
99. Mandelaris, G.A.; Rosenfeld, A.L. A novel approach to the antral sinus bone graft technique: The use of a prototype cutting guide for precise outlining of the lateral wall. A case report. *Int. J. Periodontics Restor. Dent.* **2008**, *28*, 569–575.
100. Pistilli, R.; Canullo, L.; Pesce, P.; Pistilli, V.; Caponio, V.C.A.; Sbricoli, L. Guided implant surgery and sinus lift in severely resorbed maxillae: A retrospective clinical study with up to 10 years of follow-up. *J. Dent.* **2022**, *121*, 104137. [CrossRef]
101. Strbac, G.D.; Giannis, K.; Schnappauf, A.; Bertl, K.; Stavropoulos, A.; Ulm, C. Guided Lateral Sinus Lift Procedure Using 3-Dimensionally Printed Templates for a Safe Surgical Approach: A Proof-of-Concept Case Report. *J. Oral Maxillofac. Surg.* **2020**, *78*, 1529–1537. [CrossRef]
102. Osman, A.H.; Mansour, H.; Atef, M.; Hakam, M. Computer guided sinus floor elevation through lateral window approach with simultaneous implant placement. *Clin. Implant. Dent. Relat. Res.* **2017**, *20*, 137–143. [CrossRef]
103. Pozzi, A.; Moy, P.K. Minimally Invasive Transcrestal Guided Sinus Lift (TGSL): A Clinical Prospective Proof-of-Concept Cohort Study up to 52 Months. *Clin. Implant. Dent. Relat. Res.* **2013**, *16*, 582–593. [CrossRef]
104. An, X.; Lee, C.; Fang, Y.; Choi, B. Immediate nonfunctional loading of implants placed simultaneously using computer-guided flapless maxillary crestal sinus augmentation with bone morphogenetic protein-2/collagen matrix. *Clin. Implant. Dent. Relat. Res.* **2019**, *21*, 1054–1061. [CrossRef]
105. Mauer, R.G.; Shadrav, A.; Dashti, M. Static Surgical Guides and Dynamic Navigation in Implant Surgery. In *Navigation in Oral and Maxillofacial Surgery: Applications, Advances, and Limitations*; Parhiz, S.A., James, J.N., Ghasemi, S., Amirzade-Iranaq, M.H., Eds.; Springer International Publishing: Cham, Switzerland, 2022; pp. 135–150.
106. Block, M.S.; Emery, R.W.; Cullum, D.R.; Sheikh, A. Implant Placement Is More Accurate Using Dynamic Navigation. *J. Oral Maxillofac. Surg.* **2017**, *75*, 1377–1386. [CrossRef]
107. Wu, B.-Z.; Ma, F.-F.; Sun, F. Analysis of the accuracy of a dynamic navigation system when performing dental implant surgery with transcrestal sinus floor elevation: A pilot study. *J. Dent. Sci.* **2023**. [CrossRef]
108. Blake, F.; Blessmann, M.; Pohlenz, P.; Heiland, M. A new imaging modality for intraoperative evaluation of sinus floor augmentation. *Int. J. Oral Maxillofac. Surg.* **2008**, *37*, 183–185. [CrossRef] [PubMed]
109. Dellavia, C.; Speroni, S.; Pellegrini, G.; Gatto, A.; Maiorana, C. A New Method to Evaluate Volumetric Changes in Sinus Augmentation Procedure. *Clin. Implant. Dent. Relat. Res.* **2013**, *16*, 684–690. [CrossRef] [PubMed]
110. Diserens, V.; Mericske, E.; Mericske-Stern, R. Radiographic Analysis of the Transcrestal Sinus Floor Elevation: Short-Term Observations. *Clin. Implant. Dent. Relat. Res.* **2005**, *7*, 70–78. [CrossRef]
111. Gray, C.F.; Redpath, T.W.; Bainton, R.; Smith, F.W. Magnetic resonance imaging assessment of a sinus lift operation using reoxidised cellulose (SurgicelR) as graft material. *Clin. Oral Implant. Res.* **2001**, *12*, 526–530. [CrossRef]

112. Hallman, M.; Hedin, M.; Sennerby, L.; Lundgren, S. A prospective 1-year clinical and radiographic study of implants placed after maxillary sinus floor augmentation with bovine hydroxyapatite and autogenous bone. *J. Oral Maxillofac. Surg.* **2002**, *60*, 277–284. [CrossRef]
113. Johansson, B.; Grepe, A.; Wannfors, K.; Aberg, P.; Hirsch, J.M. Volumetry of simulated bone grafts in the edentulous maxilla by computed tomography: An experimental study. *Dentomaxillofacial Radiol.* **2001**, *30*, 153–156. [CrossRef]
114. Kirmeier, R.; Arnetzl, C.; Robl, T.; Payer, M.; Lorenzoni, M.; Jakse, N. Reproducibility of volumetric measurements on maxillary sinuses. *Int. J. Oral Maxillofac. Surg.* **2011**, *40*, 195–199. [CrossRef]
115. Klijn, R.J.; Meijer, G.J.; Bronkhorst, E.M.; Jansen, J.A. Sinus Floor Augmentation Surgery Using Autologous Bone Grafts from Various Donor Sites: A Meta-Analysis of the Total Bone Volume. *Tissue Eng. Part B Rev.* **2010**, *16*, 295–303. [CrossRef]
116. Ozyuvaci, H.; Bilgiç, B.; Firatli, E. Radiologic and Histomorphometric Evaluation of Maxillary Sinus Grafting with Alloplastic Graft Materials. *J. Periodontol.* **2003**, *74*, 909–915. [CrossRef]
117. Reinert, S.; König, S.; Bremerich, A.; Eufinger, H.; Krimmel, M. Stability of bone grafting and placement of implants in the severely atrophic maxilla. *Br. J. Oral Maxillofac. Surg.* **2003**, *41*, 249–255. [CrossRef]
118. Riachi, F.; Naaman, N.; Tabarani, C.; Aboelsaad, N.; Aboushelib, M.N.; Berberi, A.; Salameh, Z. Influence of Material Properties on Rate of Resorption of Two Bone Graft Materials after Sinus Lift Using Radiographic Assessment. *Int. J. Dent.* **2012**, *2012*, 737262. [CrossRef] [PubMed]
119. Szabó, G.; Huys, L.; Coulthard, P.; Maiorana, C.; Garagiola, U.; Barabás, J.; Németh, Z.; Hrabák, K.; Suba, Z. A prospective multicenter randomized clinical trial of autogenous bone versus beta-tricalcium phosphate graft alone for bilateral sinus elevation: Histologic and histomorphometric evaluation. *Int. J. Oral Maxillofac. Implant.* **2005**, *20*, 371–381.
120. Wanschitz, F.; Figl, M.; Wagner, A.; Rolf, E. Measurement of volume changes after sinus floor augmentation with a phycogenic hydroxyapatite. *Int. J. Oral Maxillofac. Implant.* **2006**, *21*, 433–438.
121. Zijderveld, S.A.; Schulten, E.A.J.M.; Aartman, I.H.A.; ten Bruggenkate, C.M. Long-term changes in graft height after maxillary sinus floor elevation with different grafting materials: Radiographic evaluation with a minimum follow-up of 4.5 years. *Clin. Oral Implant. Res.* **2009**, *20*, 691–700. [CrossRef]
122. Hatano, N.; Shimizu, Y.; Ooya, K. A clinical long-term radiographic evaluation of graft height changes after maxillary sinus floor augmentation with a 2: 1 autogenous bone/xenograft mixture and simultaneous placement of dental implants. *Clin. Oral Implant. Res.* **2004**, *15*, 339–345. [CrossRef]
123. Hürzeler, M.B.; Kirsch, A.; Ackermann, K.L.; Quiñones, C.R. Reconstruction of the severely resorbed maxilla with dental implants in the augmented maxillary sinus: A 5-year clinical investigation. *Int. J. Oral Maxillofac. Implant.* **1996**, *11*, 466–475.
124. Galindo-Moreno, P.; Hernández-Cortés, P.; Mesa, F.; Carranza, N.; Juodžbalys, G.; Aguilar, M.; Dds, P.G.; Hernández-Cortés, P. Slow Resorption of Anorganic Bovine Bone by Osteoclasts in Maxillary Sinus Augmentation. *Clin. Implant. Dent. Relat. Res.* **2012**, *15*, 858–866. [CrossRef]
125. Kirmeier, R.; Payer, M.; Wehrschuetz, M.; Jakse, N.; Platzer, S.; Lorenzoni, M. Evaluation of three-dimensional changes after sinus floor augmentation with different grafting materials. *Clin. Oral Implant. Res.* **2008**, *19*, 366–372. [CrossRef]
126. Mazzocco, F.; Lops, D.; Gobbato, L.; Lolato, A.; Romeo, E.; Del Fabbro, M. Three-Dimensional Volume Change of Grafted Bone in the Maxillary Sinus. *Int. J. Oral Maxillofac. Implant.* **2014**, *29*, 178–184. [CrossRef]
127. Molina, A.; Sanz-Sánchez, I.; Sanz-Martín, I.; Ortiz-Vigón, A.; Sanz, M. Complications in sinus lifting procedures: Classification and management. *Periodontology 2000* **2022**, *88*, 103–115. [CrossRef]
128. Zhou, C.; Sun, S.-Z.; Lin, M.-N.; He, F.-M. Responses of Sinus Membrane and Antral Pseudocyst Following Lateral Window Sinus Augmentation with Bone Grafting: A Retrospective Study. *Int. J. Oral Maxillofac. Implant.* **2021**, *36*, 885–893. [CrossRef]
129. Jiang, X.; He, S.; Bornstein, M.M.; Wu, Y.; Ye, L.; Wang, F. Effects of different grafting materials on volumetric changes in the Schneiderian membrane following lateral maxillary sinus floor elevation: A preliminary study. *BMC Oral Health* **2023**, *23*, 102. [CrossRef]
130. Gillies, R.J.; Kinahan, P.E.; Hricak, H. Radiomics: Images Are More than Pictures, They Are Data. *Radiology* **2016**, *278*, 563–577. [CrossRef]
131. Leite, A.F.; Vasconcelos, K.D.F.; Willems, H.; Jacobs, R. Radiomics and Machine Learning in Oral Healthcare. *Proteom. Clin. Appl.* **2020**, *14*, e1900040. [CrossRef]
132. Santos, G.N.M.; da Silva, H.E.C.; Ossege, F.E.L.; Figueiredo, P.T.D.S.; Melo, N.D.S.; Stefani, C.M.; Leite, A.F. Radiomics in bone pathology of the jaws. *Dentomaxillofacial Radiol.* **2023**, *52*, 20220225. [CrossRef]

Disclaimer/Publisher's Note: The statements, opinions and data contained in all publications are solely those of the individual author(s) and contributor(s) and not of MDPI and/or the editor(s). MDPI and/or the editor(s) disclaim responsibility for any injury to people or property resulting from any ideas, methods, instructions or products referred to in the content.

diagnostics

MDPI

Article

Prevalence of Incidental Maxillary Sinus Anomalies on CBCT Scans: A Radiographic Study

Junaid Ahmed, Aditya Gupta, Nandita Shenoy *, Nanditha Sujir and Archana Muralidharan

Department of Oral Medicine and Radiology, Manipal College of Dental Sciences Mangalore, Manipal Academy of Higher Education, Manipal 575001, Karnataka, India; junaid.ahmed@manipal.edu (J.A.); adityagupta@gmail.com (A.G.); nanditha.sujir@manipal.edu (N.S.); m.archana@manipal.edu (A.M.)

* Correspondence: nandita.shenoy@manipal.edu; Tel.: +91-9901730507

Abstract: CBCT significantly impacts dental procedures and has brought significant reforms to our approach to diagnosis and treatment planning despite its limitations in differentiating soft tissues. It is an excellent imaging modality and quickly identifies sinus opacification and provides valuable insight into paranasal sinus pathologies, with considerably lower radiation exposure. The present study aimed to investigate the occurrence of maxillary sinus abnormalities in CBCT scans, identify the frequency, type, and location of these findings, and find the correlation between the distance of periapical lesions and radiographic changes in the maxillary sinus. Two examiners independently evaluated 117 patients to diagnose and classify the cases into different abnormality subtypes. The periapical lesions most closely related to the sinus were recorded. The diameters of the left and right maxillary sinus ostium and the distance of the ostium's lower border to the sinus's osseous floor were recorded. The findings were correlated with the age and gender of these patients. The present study reveals that sixty-one patients were diagnosed with mucosal thickening (52.1%). The sinus wall most affected by mucosal thickening was the maxillary sinus floor, followed by the medial and lateral walls. Of 19 patients with periapical lesions, 15 had maxillary sinus mucosal thickening, which is statistically significant ($p = 0.004$). The high occurrence of abnormalities in the maxillary sinus emphasizes the importance for the radiologist to comprehensively interpret the whole volume acquired in CBCT images, including the entire sinus. Incidental findings may be considered in the individual clinical context of signs and symptoms, reducing the risk of overestimating the real impact of radiographic findings.

Keywords: cone beam computed tomography; maxillary sinus; pathology; polyps; well being

1. Introduction

Incidental findings in the maxillary sinus are unexpected or unintended discoveries that are not directly related to the primary reason for conducting a cone beam computed tomography (CBCT) scan for dental imaging [1,2]. CBCT scans are often used in dentistry to visualize the oral and maxillofacial structures, including the teeth, jawbones, and surrounding tissues. However, due to the detailed nature of CBCT imaging, it is not uncommon to identify other anatomical structures or conditions [3–5]. Here are some examples of incidental findings that might be identified in the maxillary sinus during a CBCT scan taken for dental imaging:

Sinusitis: Inflammation or infection of the maxillary sinus can be observed on a CBCT scan, showing changes in the sinus lining and the presence of fluid or air–fluid levels [6].

Retention Cysts: These are fluid-filled sacs that can develop within the sinus due to blocked ducts. They are usually benign and may not require immediate treatment.

Polyps: Nasal or sinus polyps, which are non-cancerous growths, can sometimes be identified incidentally. They may cause congestion or sinus issues [7].

Mucous Retention Pseudocysts: These benign cystic lesions occur when the mucus becomes trapped in a blocked sinus cavity, causing the sinus lining to expand.

Anatomical Variations: Some people may have anatomical variations in the maxillary sinus, such as septa (dividing walls) or accessory ostia (additional openings). These variations are usually harmless [8].

Tumors or Masses: Rarely, tumors or masses might be identified incidentally within the maxillary sinus. Further evaluation is needed to determine such a finding's nature and potential implications.

Foreign Bodies: Foreign objects that have entered the maxillary sinus, such as dental materials or fragments, might be detected during imaging [9].

Bone Pathologies: Conditions like fibrous dysplasia, osteomas, or cysts in the maxillary sinus area can be identified incidentally [10].

Dental Pathologies: Infections originating from dental roots can sometimes spread to the maxillary sinus, leading to sinus infections or abscesses. As a result, conditions affecting the maxillary sinuses can imitate dental problems and vice versa [11]. Radiographs are frequently used to diagnose diseases of the maxillary sinus, ranging from conventional 2D imaging, like panoramic radiograph and posteroanterior views of sinuses, to the more advanced 3D imaging modalities, like cone beam computed tomography (CBCT), computed tomography (CT), and magnetic resonance imaging (MRI). The multiplanar images acquired by CBCT allow radiologists to inspect the entire volume of the acquired image and anatomic variations or abnormalities found in the image volume [12]. The maxillary sinus area is usually within the imaging field when CBCT is indicated for dental implant site assessment or periapical pathologies [13]. Hence, maxillofacial radiologists frequently view the incidental findings in the maxillary sinus area and can assess the prevalence, which can be incidental, benign, or detrimental to the treatment plan.

It is important to note that not all incidental findings require immediate intervention. The clinical significance of each finding depends on factors such as the patient's symptoms, medical history, and the nature of the finding itself. If an incidental finding is identified, the dental or medical professional may recommend further evaluation or referral to an appropriate specialist, such as an ear, nose, and throat (ENT) surgeon.

In a study by Cha et al. [14], using CBCT examinations, the abnormalities found were signs of sinusitis (7.5%), retention cysts (3.5%), and polypoid mucosal thickening (2.3%). In another study, the prevalence of flat mucosal thickening ranged from 23.7% to 38.1%, that of polypoid mucosal thickening ranged from 6.5% to19.4%, signs of acute sinusitis made up 3.6%, and partial and total opacification made up 12% and 7%, respectively [1].

The inability of a general dentist to detect incidental abnormalities in the maxillary sinus despite being visible in the CBCT volume is often due to their limited experience in interpreting volumetric images and their failure to conduct a thorough visual examination of the entire image [15]. The European Academy of DentoMaxilloFacial Radiology (EADMFR) and the American Academy of Oral and Maxillofacial Radiology (AAOMR) outline that an oral and maxillofacial radiologist should review and interpret the entire volume regardless of the region of interest [16].

The present study was undertaken to record the prevalence of incidental maxillary sinus abnormalities in CBCT scans, recognize the frequency, type, and location of these findings, and correlate the distance between the periapical lesions and the presence of any inflammatory changes in the maxillary sinus.

2. Materials and Methods

The retrospective study was conducted in the Department of Oral Medicine and Radiology, Manipal College of Dental Sciences, Mangalore. After receiving approval from the Institutional Ethical Committee, MAHE/MCODSMLR/198/2021, a statistician was consulted. Considering the power of the study to be 80%, with an alpha of 5%, the corresponding z value is $Z = -1.95996398454005$. Using the formula $n = (Z\alpha/2d)2\ p(1 - p)$ with the minimum percentage difference deemed clinically significant at 8.1%, the sample size required was 117 for the study. It was advised to include 117 patient scans.

Detailed information regarding age, gender, facial asymmetry, trauma, and history of upper respiratory infections was obtained from the patients' past medical records. Large FOV CBCT scans were included in the study, extended from the roof of the orbits inferiorly to at least the second cervical vertebrae of the patients above 18. Scans of edentulous patients, patients referred exclusively for maxillary sinus abnormalities, young patients with incomplete sinus development, low-resolution images, and those with metallic artifacts that impaired sinus visualization were excluded.

The CBCT images were obtained using standard exposure parameters and patient positioning protocols (field of view= 17 × 10 cm, resolution = 0.16 mm, 80–84 kvp, 10–12 mA) with a CBCT unit (Planmeca promax 3D Mid, Helsinki, Finland). Romexis version 4.6.2 software (Planmeca, Helsinki, Finland) was used. The exposure parameters were standardized for all the patients. The CBCT scans had panoramic reconstruction and multiplanar reformation views, i.e., axial, sagittal, and coronal planes. Two examiners who have completed their master's degrees in oral radiology assessed all images to diagnose and classify them into different abnormality subtypes. In the case of a discrepancy between two observers, a third examiner intervened, and a consensus on the radiologic impression was obtained. The presence or absence of sinus abnormalities was identified using a yes/no scale. The radiology reports followed a consistent format and contained a listing of all radiographic findings used to tabulate the data in this study using Microsoft Excel.

1. Increased or decreased dimension of the sinus;
2. Radiographic density changes in the cortical bone of the sinus;
3. Partial or complete opacification of the sinus cavity;
4. Increased thickening of the mucosa greater than 3 mm;
5. Congenital changes (aplasia and hypoplasia);
6. Inflammatory lesions like polyps;
7. Fracture lines.

The patients were divided into the following age groups: (1) <20; (2) 21–30; (3) 31–40; (4) 41–50; (5) 51–60; (6) 61 years and above.

The locations of the diagnosed abnormalities were recorded as affecting either the anterior, posterior, inferior, superior, lateral, or medial walls of the sinus based on the method by Nishimura and Iizuka [17]. The presence of periapical lesions in the upper posterior teeth was recorded. The lesions' proximity to the sinus wall floor was classified using the method followed by Oberli et al. [18]. They were classified as Class I (near the sinus floor), Class II (in contact with the sinus floor), or Class III (overlapping with the sinus floor). A periapical lesion was recorded when the lamina dura was imperceptible or had an irregular appearance and when there was a radiolucency indicating bone destruction around the root apex. The connection between the teeth affected by periapical infection and the sinus floor was investigated through sagittal and coronal reconstructions. The findings were categorized as follows:

1. No contact between the root apex and the maxillary sinus existed.
2. It appeared that one of the tooth roots was either touching the sinus floor or extending into the maxillary sinus. One of the tooth roots was either touching the sinus floor or extending into the maxillary sinus.
3. More than two teeth appeared to be in contact with the sinus floor or protruded into the maxillary sinus.

Based on the above criteria, teeth with periapical lesions were graded based on the anatomic relationship as 1, 2, or 3, as described earlier. Because not all roots have the same spatial connection with the maxillary sinus, the root and/or the periapical lesion nearest the sinus floor was continuously recorded. Only the lesion most closely related to the sinus was recorded in cases of multiple periapical lesions near the sinuses. The above findings were all correlated with the age and gender of the patient.

Statistical Analysis

A Chi-square test was used to compare the patterns with gender and age using SPSS version 17.0 (SPSS Inc., Chicago, IL, USA) for data analysis. The results are considered significant at a p-value of <0.05.

3. Results

A total of 55 patients (47%) were male, and 62 (53%) were female. The most common indication for CBCT scans was dental implant site assessment, surgical planning, orthodontic scans, TMJ dysfunction, suspected oral malignancies, and trauma.

A total of 68 patients had pathologic findings in one or both sinuses, such as mucosal thickening, odontogenic cysts, fracture, hypoplasia, and bone lesions (58.1%) (Figures 1–4). Of the 55 male patients, 33 had pathologies, like oroantral communication and inflammatory cysts in either sinus, whereas only 35 of the 62 scans of the female patients revealed radiographically abnormal findings in either sinus. The difference between the male and female patients was insignificant (Table 1).

Patients in their sixth decade of life showed a slightly higher prevalence of pathologic findings in the maxillary sinus, which was statistically significant (p = 0.017) (Table 2).

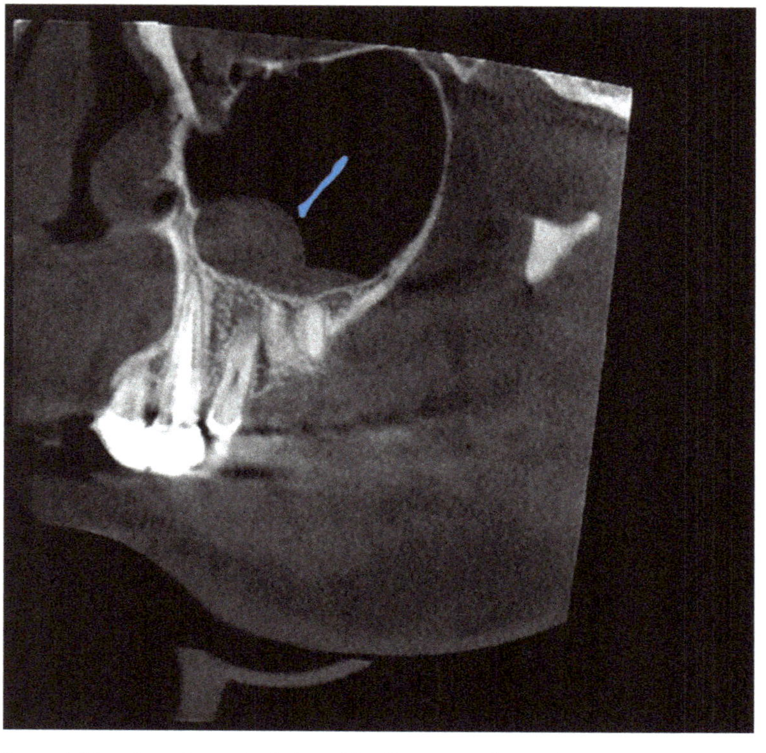

Figure 1. View from the sagittal plane. The Blue arrow shows shows a thickening of the mucous boundaries of the maxillary sinuses.

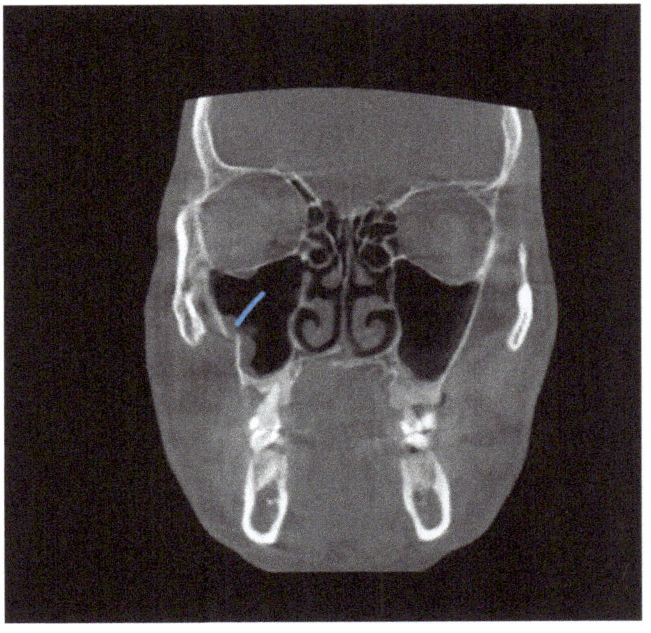

Figure 2. View from the coronal plane. The Blue arrow shows a fracture line along the lateral wall of the maxillary sinuses.

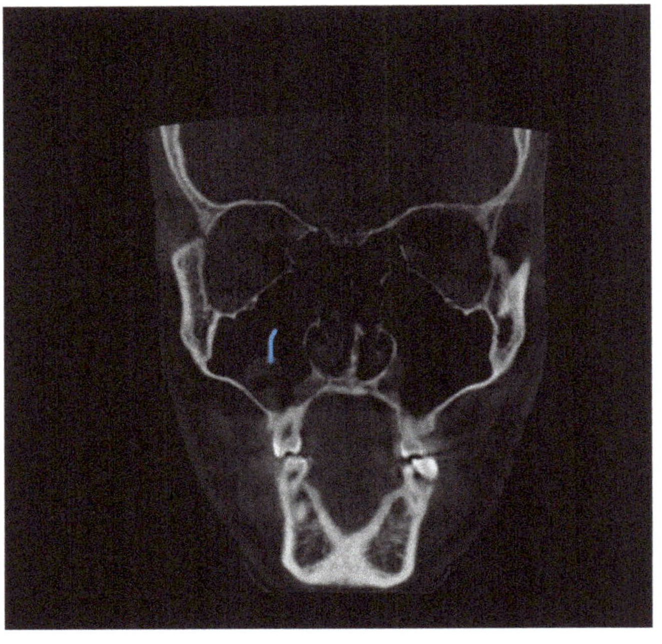

Figure 3. View from the coronal plane. The Blue arrow shows a polypoid growth along the floor of the right maxillary sinuses.

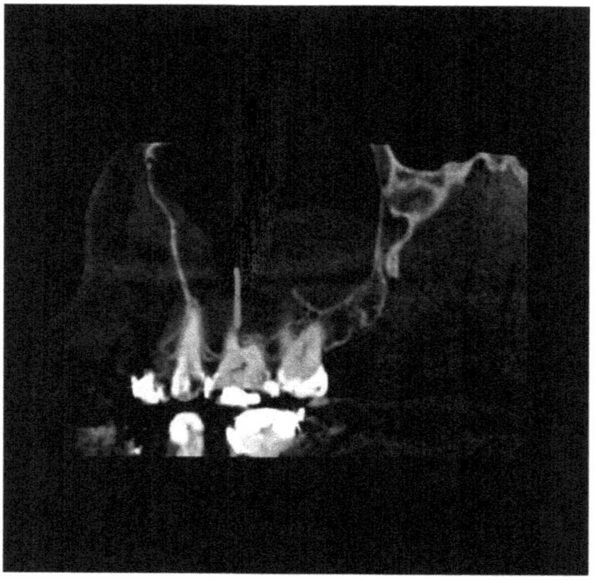

Figure 4. View from the sagittal plane. The Blue arrow shows the close proximity of the periapical lesion in the maxillary molar and the associated sinus wall thickening.

Table 1. Sex-wise distribution of pathologies.

		SEX		Chi-Square	p-Value
		F	M		
		Count	Count		
Abnormality in sinus	NO	27	22	0.1510	0.6980
	YES	35	33		
Mucosal thickening	NO	31	25	0.2410	0.6230
	YES	31	30		
Odontogenic cyst	NO	59	53	0.1030	0.7480
	YES	3	2		
Odontogenic tumor	NO	62	55	0	0
	YES	0	0		
Bone lesion	NO	61	54	0.0070	0.9320
	YES	1	1		
Fracture	NO	61	54	0.0070	0.9320
	YES	1	1		
Hypoplasia	NO	60	54	0.2310	0.6310
	YES	2	1		
Periapical lesion	NO	50	48	0.9410	0.3320
	YES	12	7		
Periapical grade	1	5	5	2.4040	0.3010
	2	5	1		
	3	1	0		

Table 2. Age-wise distribution of pathologies.

		AGE												Chi-Square	p-Value
		≤20		21–30		31–40		41–50		51–60		>61			
		Count	Column N %	Count	Column N %	Count	Column N %	Count	Column N %	Count	Column N %	Count	Column N %		
Abnormality in sinus	NO	15	46.9%	7	30.4%	6	54.5%	4	26.7%	14	70.0%	3	18.8%	13.7310	0.017
	YES	17	53.1%	16	69.6%	5	45.5%	11	73.3%	6	30.0%	13	81.3%		
Mucosal thickening	NO	16	50.0%	10	43.5%	6	54.5%	6	40.0%	14	70.0%	4	25.0%	8.0830	0.1520
	YES	16	50.0%	13	56.5%	5	45.5%	9	60.0%	6	30.0%	12	75.0%		
Odontogenic cyst	NO	31	96.9%	21	91.3%	11	100.0%	14	93.3%	20	100.0%	15	93.8%	2.9490	0.7080
	YES	1	3.1%	2	8.7%	0	0.0%	1	6.7%	0	0.0%	1	6.3%		
Odontogenic tumor	NO	32	100.0%	23	100.0%	11	100.0%	15	100.0%	20	100.0%	16	100.0%	00	0.00
	YES	0	0.0%	0	0.0%	0	0.0%	0	0.0%	0	0.0%	0	0.0%		
Bone lesion	NO	32	100.0%	22	95.7%	11	100.0%	14	93.3%	20	100.0%	16	100.0%	4.5210	0.4770
	YES	0	0.0%	1	4.3%	0	0.0%	1	6.7%	0	0.0%	0	0.0%		
Fracture	NO	32	100.0%	22	95.7%	11	100.0%	14	93.3%	20	100.0%	16	100.0%	4.5210	0.4770
	YES	0	0.0%	1	4.3%	0	0.0%	1	6.7%	0	0.0%	0	0.0%		
Opacification	NO	31	96.9%	23	100.0%	11	100.0%	15	100.0%	19	95.0%	15	93.8%	2.6750	0.7500
	YES	1	3.1%	0	0.0%	0	0.0%	0	0.0%	1	5.0%	1	6.3%		
Periapical lesion	NO	26	81.3%	19	82.6%	10	90.9%	11	73.3%	18	90.0%	14	87.5%	2.5200	0.7730
	YES	6	18.8%	4	17.4%	1	9.1%	4	26.7%	2	10.0%	2	12.5%		
Periapical grade	1	2	50.0%	2	50.0%	0	0.0%	4	100.0%	0	0.0%	2	100.0%	12.8920	0.2300
	2	2	50.0%	1	25.0%	1	100.0%	0	0.0%	2	100.0%	0	0.0%		
	3	0	0.0%	1	25.0%	0	0.0%	0	0.0%	0	0.0%	0	0.0%		

A total of 61 patients were diagnosed with mucosal thickening (52.1%). The sinus wall most affected by mucosal thickening was the maxillary sinus floor, followed by the medial and lateral walls of the maxillary sinus. Of the 19 patients with odontogenic conditions causing periapical lesions, 15 had maxillary sinus mucosal thickening, and the relation was statistically significant (p = 0.004). The odontogenic cyst was diagnosed in five patients (4.3%), while a sinus wall fracture was recorded in two patients (1.7%). Maxillary sinus hypoplasia was diagnosed in three patients (2.6%). We did not observe any significant difference between the periapical grade and the occurrence of maxillary sinusitis, even though we had five cases of Grades 2 and 3, which meant that in five cases, there was a periapical region close to the maxillary sinus, which could induce a change in the latter. The frequency of the pathologies is represented in Figure 5.

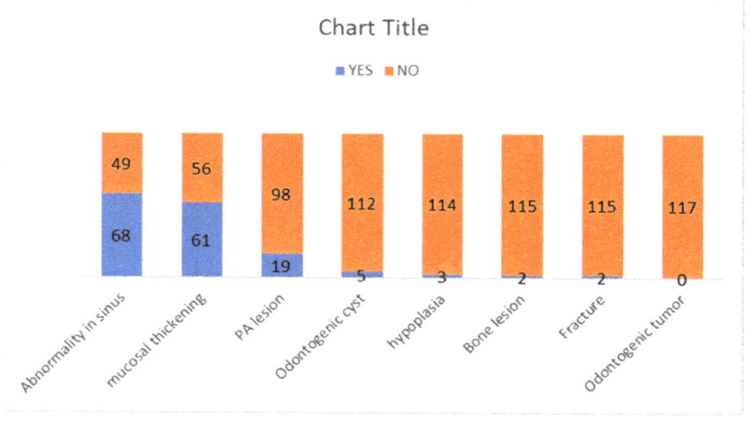

Figure 5. The frequency of the pathologies seen as incidental findings in the maxillary sinus.

4. Discussion

CBCT, a 3D imaging modality, could be of clinical value in screening and planning paranasal surgery. Studies have reported the valuable application of CBCT for intraoperative imaging of the paranasal sinus [19]. One of the benefits of applying CBCT for imaging of the paranasal sinuses could be the lower dose compared to CT imaging. Moreover, CBCT delivers an isotropic volume resolution, facilitating the diagnosis of delicate structures in multiplanar reconstructions [20]. This study assessed the prevalence of incidental findings in the maxillary sinus using cone beam computerized tomography scans of patients referred to the department. The results show a high prevalence of abnormalities in the maxillary sinus, highlighting the need for thoroughly examining the entire volume of the CBCT image, which includes the maxillary sinus and its associated regions.

Many studies have acknowledged that interpreting CBCT images necessitates familiarity with the anatomy of the area being investigated, comprehension of the spatial relationships within the image volume, a deep understanding of the potential diseases, anatomical variations, and abnormalities that impact the maxillofacial region, and the ability to formulate a differential diagnosis with expertise [21].

For dental implant site assessment in the maxilla, the configuration and status of the maxillary sinus are essential to assess the available amount of bone. If a sinus lift is indicated, the visualization is helpful because the success rate of sinus lift procedures is crucially dependent on the configuration and status of the maxillary sinus [22]. Any disease arising from dental or dentoalveolar structures could damage the floor of the maxillary sinus, leading to sinusitis, known as odontogenic maxillary sinusitis (OMS). The maxillary sinus and the associated teeth are better revealed in CBCT than in periapical radiography [23,24].

Several studies have reported significant variability in the prevalence of incidental findings in the maxillary sinuses of asymptomatic subjects in multiplanar images [25–27]. CT is considered the gold standard for adequate maxillary sinus imaging because of its high resolution and ability to discern bone and soft tissue and detect sinus inflammation in approximately 30% of cases [28]. A CBCT study reported a prevalence of 24.6% to 56.3% [29], whereas our research saw incidental abnormalities in 68.3%. Discrepancies in these variations may be due to several factors, such as dissimilarities in the sampling criteria, variations in image interpretation, and the diagnostic criteria used.

Our study covered a wide range of age distribution; it did not include patients under 12 years since the formation of their maxillary sinus is still incomplete, and specific abnormalities such as mucosal thickening and opacification are common findings in early childhood and not indicative of sinus disease. The most detected abnormality was mucosal thickening, observed in 52.1% of cases, especially among individuals under 20 and between 20 and 30 years old. A study carried out by Rege [30] also had a similar finding, where mucosal thickening was associated with irritation, such as odontogenic pathology or allergic phenomena. Nonvital posterior maxillary teeth, periodontal abscesses, retained roots, embedded, or impacted teeth, extensively carious teeth, and oroantral fistulae could be etiological factors in pathologies of odontogenic origin causing mucosal thickening [16].

Correlation between periapical lesions and maxillary sinusitis: There is a potential correlation between periapical lesions and maxillary sinusitis due to their proximity to the upper jaw [31]. The roots of the upper back teeth (molars and premolars) are situated close to the maxillary sinus floor. An advanced periapical infection in these teeth can erode the bone, separating the root tip from the sinus, and creating a pathway for disease to spread from the tooth's root into the sinus cavity. This can lead to sinusitis and dental symptoms [32]. An infection from a periapical lesion can sometimes extend into the maxillary sinus, causing sinusitis symptoms. Conversely, maxillary sinusitis can sometimes cause referred pain to the upper back teeth, making it difficult to pinpoint the exact source of the discomfort. Not all cases of periapical lesions lead to maxillary sinusitis, and not all cases of maxillary sinusitis are caused by dental infections [33]. Proper diagnosis and treatment by dental and medical professionals are crucial to effectively differentiate and manage these conditions.

Research has demonstrated that periapical lesions close to or linked with the sinus floor can heighten the possibility of sinus infections. Moreover, more significant apical lesions can lead to an increase in the maxillary sinus and mucosal thickness. However, our study did not reveal any incidental discovery despite encountering five cases where the mucosal floor was near the root apices [34,35].

A study by Nurbakhsh et al. [36] found that the sinus wall thickening increased as the distance between the tooth apex or lesion and the maxillary sinuses decreased. Similarly, it was reported by Shanbhag et al. and Goller-Bulut et al. The current study did not document such findings nor find any correlation between apical proximity to the maxillary sinus and the age of the study subjects [37,38].

As a part of the multidisciplinary approach, it is recommended that a dentist and an ENT surgeon work as a team to provide an accurate diagnosis and appropriate treatment on time. The proximity between the maxillary molar roots associated with periapical lesions and the sinus floor could influence maxillary sinus irritation [27]. When periapical lesions were present, the anatomic relationship was ranked between 1 and 3, as described earlier. Because not all roots have the same spatial connection with the maxillary sinus, the heart or the periapical lesion nearest the sinus floor was continuously recorded.

Our study demonstrates a significant relationship between periapical lesions and sinus pathology ($p = 0.04$). The lower sinus wall was the most affected location within the sinus, which suggests possible odontogenic involvement [27]. The results of our study correlate with the study by Hauman et al. [27], who demonstrated a positive correlation between periapical lesions and sinus opacification.

Odontogenic cysts were the second most frequently found inflammatory abnormality (4.3%). This result is comparable to the findings of Bosio et al. [39] and Rhodus NL [29]. These studies examined general dental patients using plain panoramic radiography and reported a prevalence ranging from 1.4% to 9.6%.

The third most frequent finding was sinus opacification, observed in six patients. The deviated nasal septum was observed in 6.3% of patients; this finding is consistent with Smith et al. [40], who found that 19.4% of their patients had a deviated septum, and 50.0% had mucosal thickening and sinus opacification, which is consistent with maxillary sinusitis.

Considering the clinical implications of sinus inflammation when installing dental implants, particularly in patients with nasal septum deviation, is essential [23,24]. It is crucial to carefully assess the presence or absence of opacifications in the maxillary sinus. Opacification, which refers to clouding the sinuses, was not a finding in our study. However, it is essential to note that opacification can also result from other abnormalities such as mechanical trauma, barotraumas, and hemorrhage. While inflammation is the most likely cause, it is essential to rule out other possibilities, such as fungal sinusitis or neoplastic disease.

Raghav M et al. [41] reported that opacification could even be found in asymptomatic patients as an incidental finding in 67% of cases. Chen et al. [42] found that in cases of unilateral opacification, there was a 5.1% incidence of malignancy, a 10.4% incidence of benign tumors, and a 29.3% incidence of fungal disease. In a separate study, Kaplan et al. [43] found that patients who underwent endoscopic sinus surgery had a high incidence of mucoceles and nasal polyposis in cases of complete unilateral opacification. Additionally, in a review of 1118 CT scans of the maxillary sinus, Ahsan et al. [44] found that 28 of these had complete opacification, with 12 of these patients being further diagnosed with neoplastic disease.

One limitation of this study is the limited sample size and the need for prospective studies. We also recommend a multidisciplinary approach toward the management of such incidental findings. The present study stresses the importance of radiologists being alert and observing alterations that may not be related to the reasons for the initial examination. It is also important to note that incidental findings on radiographs should be assessed clinically as a part of proactive patient care.

5. Conclusions

The high occurrence of incidental findings in the maxillary sinus emphasizes the importance for dentomaxillofacial radiologists to comprehensively interpret the whole volume acquired in CBCT images, including the entire sinus, while analyzing the images of routine patients. Two-dimensional imaging techniques suffer from the superimposition of anatomic structures, making the documentation of incidental findings in the maxillary sinus difficult. Incidental findings may be considered in the individual clinical context of signs and symptoms, reducing the risk of overestimating the real impact of radiographic findings.

6. Patents

No patents have been filed from this study.

Author Contributions: J.A. and N.S. (Nandita Shenoy)—Substantial contributions to the conception and design of the work; the acquisition, analysis, and interpretation of data for the work; drafting the work or revising it critically for important intellectual content; final approval of the version to be published; and agreement to be accountable for all aspects of the work in ensuring that questions related to the accuracy or integrity of any part of the work are appropriately investigated and resolved. A.G., N.S. (Nanditha Sujir) and A.M.—Drafting the work and revising it critically for important intellectual content; final approval of the version to be published; and agreement to be accountable for all aspects of the work in ensuring that questions related to the accuracy or integrity of any part of the work are appropriately investigated and resolved. All authors have read and agreed to the published version of the manuscript.

Funding: This research received no external funding.

Institutional Review Board Statement: This study was conducted in accordance with the Declaration of Helsinki and approved by the Institutional Review Board (or Ethics Committee) of MCODS Mangalore (protocol code 14142).

Informed Consent Statement: Informed consent was obtained from all subjects involved in the study.

Data Availability Statement: Data supporting reported results can be found, in preprints of this journal including the archived datasets analyzed or generated during the study.

Conflicts of Interest: The authors declare no conflict of interest.

References

1. Binshabaib, M.; Alharthi, S.S.; Alkraida, R.; Aljared, S.; Alshami, A.; Mansour, S. Incidental findings in maxillary sinus area on cone-beam-computed-tomographic-scans: A retrospective study with emphasis on gender and ethnicity. *Saudi Dent. J.* **2021**, *33*, 184–187. [CrossRef] [PubMed]
2. Aktuna Belgin, C.; Colak, M.; Adiguzel, O.; Akkus, Z.; Orhan, K. Three-dimensional evaluation of maxillary sinus volume in different age and sex groups using CBCT. *Eur. Arch. Otorhinolaryngol.* **2019**, *276*, 1493–1499. [CrossRef] [PubMed]
3. Al-Rawi, B.; Hassan, B.; Vandenberge, B.; Jacobs, R. Accuracy assessment of three-dimensional surface reconstructions of teeth from cone beam computed tomography scans. *J. Oral Rehabil.* **2010**, *37*, 352–358. [CrossRef]
4. Alsufyani, N.A. Cone beam computed tomography incidental findings of the cervical spine and clivus: Retrospective analysis and review of the literature. *Oral Surg. Oral Med. Oral Pathol. Oral Radiol.* **2017**, *123*, e197–e217. [CrossRef] [PubMed]
5. Avsever, H.; Gunduz, K.; Karakoc, O.; Akyol, M.; Orhan, K. Incidental findings on cone-beam computed tomographic images: Paranasal sinus findings and nasal septum variations. *Oral Radiol.* **2018**, *34*, 40–48. [CrossRef]
6. Clark, D.; Barbu, H.; Lorean, A.; Mijiritsky, E.; Levin, L. Incidental findings of implant complications on postimplantation CBCTs: A cross-sectional study. *Clin. Implant Dent. Relat. Res.* **2017**, *19*, 776–782. [CrossRef]
7. Dawood, A.; Patel, S.; Brown, J. Cone beam CT in dental practice. *Br. Dent. J.* **2009**, *207*, 23–28. [CrossRef]
8. Dief, S.; Veitz-Keenan, A.; Amintavakoli, N.; McGowan, R. A systematic review on incidental findings in cone beam computed tomography (CBCT) scans. *Dentomaxillofac. Radiol.* **2019**, *48*, 20180396. [CrossRef]
9. Edwards, R.; Alsufyani, N.; Heo, G.; Flores-Mir, C. The frequency and nature of incidental findings in large-field cone beam computed tomography scans of an orthodontic sample. *Prog. Orthod.* **2014**, *15*, 37. [CrossRef]
10. Yigit, Y.; Ayhan, H. Incidental CT Findings of Patients Who Admitted to ER Following a Traffic Accident. *Turk. J. Emerg. Med.* **2016**, *14*, 9–14. [CrossRef]
11. Migas, K.; Kozłowski, R.; Sierocka, A.; Marczak, M. Healing of Unilateral Maxillary Sinusitis by Endodontic and Periodontal Treatment of Maxillary Teeth. *Medicina* **2022**, *58*, 1302. [CrossRef] [PubMed]
12. Cağlayan, F.; Tozoğlu, U. Incidental findings in the maxillofacial region detected by cone beam CT. *Diagn. Interv. Radiol.* **2012**, *18*, 159–163.
13. Farman, A.G.; Scarfe, W.C.; van Genuchten, M. Multidimensional imaging: Immediate and imminent issues. *Compend. Contin. Educ. Dent.* **2010**, *31*, 648–651. [PubMed]
14. Cha, J.Y.; Mah, J.; Sinclair, P. Incidental findings in the maxillofacial area with 3-dimensional cone-beam imaging. *Am. J. Orthod. Dentofac. Orthop.* **2007**, *132*, 7–14. [CrossRef] [PubMed]
15. Scarfe, W.C. Incidental findings on cone beam computed tomographic images: A pandora's box? *Oral Surg. Oral Med. Oral Pathol. Oral Radiol.* **2014**, *117*, 537–540. [CrossRef]
16. Tyndall, D.A.; Price, J.B.; Tetradis, S.; Ganz, S.D.; Hildebolt, C.; Scarfe, W.C.; American Academy of Oral and Maxillofacial Radiolog. Position statement of the American Academy of Oral and Maxillofacial Radiology on selection criteria for the use of radiology in dental implantology with emphasis on cone beam computed tomography. *Oral Surg. Oral Med. Oral Pathol. Oral Radiol.* **2012**, *113*, 817–826. [CrossRef]
17. Nishimura, T.; Iizuka, T. Evaluation of the pathophysiology of odontogenic maxillary sinusitis using bone scintigraphy. *Int. J. Oral Maxillofac. Surg.* **2002**, *31*, 389–396. [CrossRef]
18. Oberli, K.; Bornstein, M.M.; Von Arx, T. Periapical surgery and the maxillary sinus: Radiographic parameters for clinical outcome. *Oral Surg. Oral. Med. Oral Pathol. Oral Radiol. Endod.* **2007**, *103*, 848–853. [CrossRef]
19. Bozdemir, E.; Gormez, O.; Yıldırım, D.; Aydogmus Erik, A. Paranasal sinus pathoses on cone beam computed tomography. *J. Istanb. Univ. Fac. Dent.* **2016**, *50*, 27–34. [CrossRef]
20. Min, C.K.; Kim, K.A. Quantitative analysis of metal artefacts of dental implant in CBCT image by correlation analysis to mi-cro-CT: A microstructural study. *Dentomaxillofac. Radiol.* **2021**, *50*, 20200365. [CrossRef]
21. Scarfe, W.C.; Levin, M.D.; Gane, D.; Farman, A.G. Use of cone beam computed tomography in endodontics. *Int. J. Dent.* **2009**, *2009*, 634567. [CrossRef] [PubMed]
22. Ulm, C.W.; Solar, P.; Krennmair, G.; Matejka, M.; Watzek, G. Incidence and suggested surgical management of septa in sinus-lift procedures. *Int. J. Oral Maxillofac. Implant.* **1995**, *10*, 462–465.

23. Little, R.E.; Long, C.M.; Loehrl, T.A.; Poetker, D.M. Odontogenic sinusitis: A review of the current literature. *Laryngoscope Investig. Otolaryngol.* **2018**, *3*, 110–114. [CrossRef] [PubMed]
24. Nair, U.P.; Nair, M.K. Maxillary sinusitis of odontogenic origin: Cone-beam volumetric computerized tomography-aided diagnosis. *Oral Surg. Oral Med. Oral Pathol. Oral Radiol. Endod.* **2010**, *110*, e53–e57. [CrossRef]
25. Madani, G.; Beale, T.J. Sinonasal inflammatory disease. *Semin. Ultrasound CT MRI* **2009**, *30*, 17–24. [CrossRef]
26. Vallo, J.; Taipale, L.S.; Huumonen, S.; Soikkonen, K.; Norblad, A. Prevalence of mucosal abnormalities of the maxillary sinus and their relationship to dental disease in panoramic radiography: Results from the Health 2000 Hearth Examination Survery. *Oral Surg. Oral Med. Oral Pahtol Oral Radiol. Endod.* **2010**, *109*, e80–e87. [CrossRef]
27. Hauman, C.H.J.; Chandler, N.P.; Tong, D.C. Endodontic implications of the maxillary sinus: A review. *Int. Endod. J.* **2002**, *35*, 127–141. [CrossRef]
28. Noorian, V.; Motaghi, A. Assessment of the Diagnostic Accuracy of Limited CT Scan of Paranasal Sinuses in the Identification of Sinusitis. *Iran. Red Crescent Med. J.* **2012**, *14*, 709–712. [CrossRef]
29. Rhodus, N.L. The prevalence and clinical significance of maxillary sinus mucous retention cysts in a general clinic population. *Ear Nose Throat J.* **1990**, *69*, 82–87.
30. Rege, I.C.; Sousa, T.O.; Leles, C.R.; Mendonça, E.F. Occurrence of maxillary sinus abnormalities detected by cone beam CT in asymptomatic patients. *BMC Oral Health* **2012**, *12*, 30. [CrossRef]
31. Ince Yusufoglu, S.; Hasanoglu Erbasar, G.N.; Gülen, O. Evaluation of the effect of periapical lesions and other odontogenic conditions on maxillary sinus mucosal thickness characteristics and mucosal appearance: A CBCT study. *J. Dent. Res. Dent. Clin. Dent. Prospect.* **2021**, *15*, 163–171. [CrossRef] [PubMed]
32. Vestin Fredriksson, M.; Öhman, A.; Flygare, L.; Tano, K. When maxillary sinusitis does not heal: Findings on CBCT scans of the sinuses with a particular focus on the occurrence of odontogenic causes of maxillary sinusitis. *Laryngoscope Investig. Otolaryngol.* **2017**, *2*, 442–446. [CrossRef] [PubMed]
33. Dumitrescu, A.; Martu, M.-A.; Nemtoi, A.; Sirghe, A.; Chelaru, L.; Tatarciuc, D.; Dumitrescu, A.-M.; Haba, D. Association between Cone-Beam Computed Tomography and Histological and Immunohistochemical Features in Periapical Lesions Correlated with Thickened Maxillary Sinus Mucosa. *Medicina* **2021**, *57*, 840. [CrossRef]
34. Lu, Y.; Liu, Z.; Zhang, L.; Zhou, X.; Zheng, Q.; Duan, X.; Zheng, G.; Wang, H.; Huang, D. Associations between maxillary sinus mucosal thickening and apical periodontitis using cone-beam computed tomography scanning: A retrospective study. *J. Endod.* **2012**, *38*, 1069–1074. [CrossRef]
35. Sheikhi, M.; Jafari Pozve, N.; Khorrami, L. Using cone beam computed tomography to detect the relationship between the periodontal bone loss and mucosal thickening of the maxillary sinus. *Dent. Res. J.* **2014**, *11*, 495–501.
36. Nurbakhsh, B.; Friedman, S.; Kulkarni, G.V.; Basrani, B.; Lam, E. Resolution of maxillary sinus mucositis after endodontic treatment of maxillary teeth with apical periodontitis: A cone-beam computed tomography pilot study. *J. Endod.* **2011**, *37*, 1504–1511. [CrossRef] [PubMed]
37. Shanbhag, S.; Karnik, P.; Shirke, P.; Shanbhag, V. Association between periapical lesions and maxillary sinus mucosal thickening: A retrospective cone-beam computed tomographic study. *J. Endod.* **2013**, *39*, 853–857. [CrossRef]
38. Goller-Bulut, D.; Sekerci, A.E.; Köse, E.; Sisman, Y. Cone beam computed tomographic analysis of maxillary premolars and molars to detect the relationship between periapical and marginal bone loss and mucosal thickness of maxillary sinus. *Med. Oral Patol. Oral Cir. Bucal* **2015**, *20*, e572–e579. [CrossRef]
39. Bósio, J.A.; Tanaka, O.; Rovigatti, E.; Gruner, S.K. The incidence of maxillary sinus retention cysts in orthodontic patients. *World J. Orthod.* **2009**, *10*, e7–e8.
40. Smith, K.D.; Edwards, P.C.; Saini, T.S.; Norton, N.S. The prevalence of concha bullosa and nasal septal deviation and their relationship to maxillary sinusitis by volumetric tomography. *Int. J. Dent.* **2010**, *2010*, 404982. [CrossRef]
41. Raghav, M.; Karjodkar, F.R.; Sontakke, S.; Sansare, K. Prevalence of incidental maxillary sinus pathologies in dental patients on cone-beam computed tomographic images. *Contemp. Clin. Dent.* **2014**, *5*, 361–365. [CrossRef] [PubMed]
42. Chen, H.J.; Chen, H.S.; Chang, Y.L.; Huang, Y.C. Complete unilateral maxillary sinus opacity in computed tomography. *J. Formos. Med. Assoc.* **2010**, *109*, 709–715. [CrossRef] [PubMed]
43. Kaplan, B.A.; Kountakis, S.E. Diagnosis and pathology of unilateral maxillary sinus opacification with or without evidence of contralateral disease. *Laryngoscope* **2004**, *114*, 981–985. [CrossRef] [PubMed]
44. Ahsan, F.; El-Hakim, H.; Ah-See, K.W. Unilateral opacification of paranasal sinus CT scans. *Otolaryngol. Head Neck Surg.* **2005**, *133*, 178–180. [CrossRef]

Disclaimer/Publisher's Note: The statements, opinions and data contained in all publications are solely those of the individual author(s) and contributor(s) and not of MDPI and/or the editor(s). MDPI and/or the editor(s) disclaim responsibility for any injury to people or property resulting from any ideas, methods, instructions or products referred to in the content.

diagnostics

Article

Augmented Reality-Guided Apicoectomy Based on Maxillofacial CBCT Scans

Bernhard Remschmidt [1,2], Marcus Rieder [1,2], Christina Gsaxner [3], Jan Gaessler [1,2], Michael Payer [2] and Juergen Wallner [1,*]

1 Division of Oral and Maxillofacial Surgery, Department of Dental Medicine and Oral Health, Medical University of Graz, 8036 Graz, Austria
2 Division of Oral Surgery and Orthodontics, Department of Dental Medicine and Oral Health, Medical University of Graz, 8010 Graz, Austria
3 Institute of Computer Graphics and Vision, Graz University of Technology, 8010 Graz, Austria
* Correspondence: j.wallner@medunigraz.at

Abstract: Implementation of augmented reality (AR) image guidance systems using preoperative cone beam computed tomography (CBCT) scans in apicoectomies promises to help surgeons overcome iatrogenic complications associated with this procedure. This study aims to evaluate the intraoperative feasibility and usability of HoloLens 2, an established AR image guidance device, in the context of apicoectomies. Three experienced surgeons carried out four AR-guided apicoectomies each on human cadaver head specimens. Preparation and operating times of each procedure, as well as the subjective usability of HoloLens for AR image guidance in apicoectomies using the System Usability Scale (SUS), were measured. In total, twelve AR-guided apicoectomies on six human cadaver head specimens were performed ($n = 12$). The average preparation time amounted to 162 (±34) s. The surgical procedure itself took on average 9 (±2) min. There was no statistically significant difference between the three surgeons. Quantification of the usability of HoloLens revealed a mean SUS score of 80.4 (±6.8), indicating an "excellent" usability level. In conclusion, this study implies the suitability, practicality, and simplicity of AR image guidance systems such as the HoloLens in apicoectomies and advocates their routine implementation.

Keywords: apicoectomy; endodontic surgery; root-end resection; surgery; computer-assisted; augmented reality; cone beam computed tomography

1. Introduction

Cone beam computed tomography (CBCT) was developed by Arai and colleagues in 1997 with the intention of providing a more compact modification of computed tomography (CT) scans, specifically to be used in dentistry [1]. Since then, CBCT has become an indispensable aid for diagnostics and treatment planning [2]. In addition to other indications, endodontics represent one of the main areas of clinical CBCT application [1]. Regarding the detection of periapical lesions, CBCT imaging has proven to have higher sensitivity and specificity in comparison with conventional periapical or panoramic radiographs [3]. In addition to its diagnostic value, CBCT has been incorporated in the preoperative planning of apicoectomies [4]. Using microsurgical techniques, apicoectomies have a high success rate [5,6]. Yet, there are complications that can lead to failure. Considering surgeon-dependent factors, the resection of the false root end or an injury to adjacent structures are among the most frequent complications [7]. Aiming to help surgeons avoid these complications, several computer-based solutions (e.g., intraoperative navigation systems) have been tested and introduced in the recent past [8–10]. Nevertheless, conventional image guidance has its limitations. Primarily, the surgeon has to divide their attention by focusing on a monitor and the patient simultaneously, which increases mental workload and deteriorates hand-eye coordination [11,12]. Secondly, complex three-dimensional (3D) data, such as

CBCT scans, need to be projected onto monitors in two dimensions separated from the patient by a computer workstation. Thirdly, conventionally available image guidance systems are highly expensive, industry-driven, license protected- and usually involve complex and bulky setups. In dentistry, the additional expense and effort involved in assembling a guidance system is often considered unjustified for the performed procedure [13,14].

Augmented reality (AR) has the potential to overcome these limitations. AR is a transformative technology that expands the users' understanding and awareness of their environment through the incorporation of virtual content into reality [15,16]. In the medical sector, AR offers the possibility of merging imaging data with the patient, thus enabling new dimensions of 3D visualizations. AR fundamentally diverges from virtual reality (VR) in its approach, as AR preserves the user's perceptual connection to the real world while overlaying virtual elements, whereas VR immerses the user in an entirely synthetic virtual environment, severing their sensory ties to the real world [17]. In the medical sector, AR offers the possibility of merging imaging data with the patient, thus enabling new dimensions of 3D visualizations. New perspectives for pedagogical and didactic methods arise, and real-time navigation guidance is thus made possible. Specializations in dentistry that utilize this new technology include the orthognathic section of oral surgery, oral surgery and implantology, orthodontics, and endodontics. The use of AR in these fields takes advantage of AR's ability to superimpose structures needing protection as well as target structures into the user's field of view [18–24]. The leading innovative AR device that has garnered significant attention in the healthcare domain is the HoloLens (HL) (Microsoft Corp., Redmond, WA, USA) [25].

The HL is a see-through head-mounted AR display that enables users to perceive and manipulate virtual objects within their physical environment. Compared with conventional image guidance systems, the HL circumvents the surgeons' need to branch their attention between monitor and patient, providing real 3D visualization of patient-specific image data with a stereoscopic display. It is also comparably cheap and has a very slim form factor. That said, the application of the HL in dentistry has been limited up to now. Despite the proposition of several systems for 3D visualization of dental data [26–28], the majority of these systems lack comprehensive guidance capabilities. However, the proof-of-concept HL-based dental guidance systems described by Pellegrino et al. and Song et al. still rely on external navigation systems and invasive markers, respectively [18,29]. Consequently, it is evident that the true potential of see-through AR in dentistry remains largely unexplored to date.

In the context of dental procedures involving the craniofacial region, there has been a notable development in the form of a practical image guidance system based on the HL. This system, proposed by Gsaxner et al., provides several advantages, including simplified assembly, and eliminates the need for external hardware or infrastructure [30–32]. In fact, the system is based on routinely acquired pre-interventional CT scans. From the CT scan, data about a patient's skin surface can be extracted. Then, the AR system achieves an automatic and markerless registration between the extracted skin model and the physical patient, solely by using the adeptness of the HL hardware.

The current study aims to evaluate the potential benefits of incorporating such an AR guidance system using dental CBCT scans in apicoectomy procedures.

2. Materials and Methods

Three experienced surgeons carried out four guided apicoectomies each on human cadaver head specimens to evaluate the potential benefits of an HL-based AR guidance system. Each specimen underwent a prior CBCT scan. The maxillary lateral incisor teeth, as well as the entire facial skeleton and skin surface, were segmented for visualization in AR. These data were precisely overlaid with the specimen before the surgery.

2.1. Data and Specimen Collection

The current study was carried out using tissues of human cadaver head specimens provided by the Division of Macroscopic and Clinical Anatomy at the Medical University of Graz. All cadaver specimens were preserved using Thiel's method, a high-quality embalming technique used for advanced surgical training and anatomical research purposes [33,34]. Protected by the Styrian Death and Funeral Act of 2010, permission to use post-mortem tissues was granted after undergoing an institutional review. All specimens were handled in conformity with the strict rules of the donation program of the aforementioned division. Furthermore, approval of the protocol was obtained from the institutional ethics committee (IRB00002556, re: 31-416 ex 18/19).

In order to generate an objectively comparable and standardized sample size, this study followed strict inclusion and exclusion criteria. As a first step, all specimens were screened for their eligibility using an intraoral examination performed by an experienced maxillofacial surgeon. An apicoectomy was performed on the right and left maxillary lateral incisors. The primary inclusion criterion for further involvement was anatomical integrity of the maxilla with a dentition including all maxillary incisors and canines. Further inclusion criteria were maturity of the specimens (i.e., adult age) and complete preservation of soft and hard tissues. In the following step, all included specimens underwent a standard dose CBCT scan (96 kV, 5.6 mA, exposure time 9.335 s, field of view (FOV) 23 × 27.5 mm, voxel size 0.400 mm, slice thickness 1 mm). Succeeding the CBCT scan, the application of pre-defined exclusion criteria (i.e., dental restoration material leading to artifacts in the CBCT scan causing significant overlay with the surgical field and a previously performed apicoectomy on the maxillary lateral incisors) resulted in the exclusion of further specimens from this study, as shown in Figure 1.

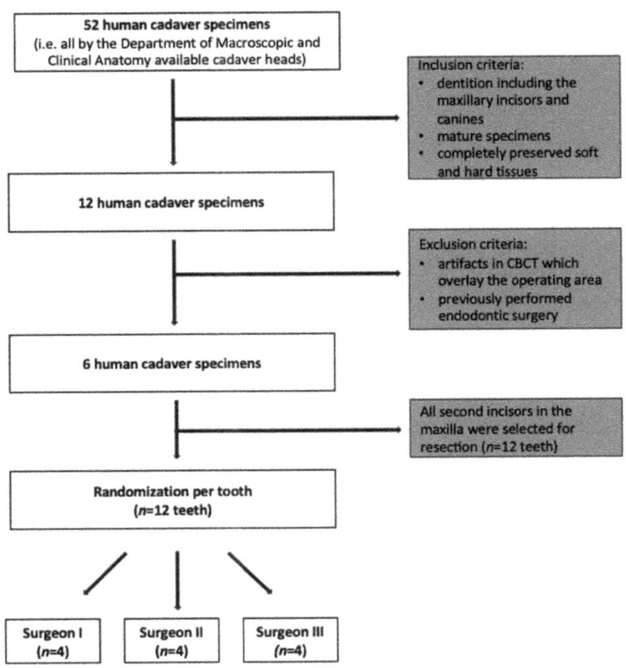

Figure 1. The flowchart illustrates the enrollment and allocation of the study design. The established high-quality preservation method by Thiel was utilized to preserve all human cadaver head specimens [33].

2.2. Augmented Reality System

An AR image guidance system based on the second version of HL (i.e., HL 2) was implemented. The HL 2 features a self-localization algorithm, which maps the surroundings of the user and localizes the device within. This enables users to position virtual content at specific locations within the mapped environment. Users can effortlessly explore said virtual objects by adjusting their viewpoint, resulting in an intuitive and immersive experience. Furthermore, the HL 2 is equipped with a time-of-flight (ToF) depth sensor, capable of capturing an exact 3D representation of the patient in the physical space. The distinct nature of human faces and the relative rigidity of facial structures can be exploited to automatically match the 3D representation of the patient captured by the HL 2 with a 3D model obtained from pre-interventional CBCT imaging. Once registered, imaging data are displayed automatically, overlaid onto the patient. The application is then controlled with a virtual user interface to alternate between different visualization modes, including 3D surface structures and planar slices. All structures are individually displayable, and their transparency and brightness can be adjusted using sliders. In the following sections, the AR system is explained in further detail.

2.2.1. Registration

Patient registration is fully automated in the system used, eliminating external navigation systems, markers, or arduous assembly procedures [31,32]. In short, it uses video frames from the HL 2 video camera, as well as depth maps from the ToF depth sensor. Using a deep learning-based, single-shot, multi-box detector [35], a bounding box around the patient's face is recognized reliably and in real time. This bounding box is mapped to the depth frame, subsequently reconstructing a point cloud representation of the patient's face with the application of inverse perspective transformation. The point cloud is matched to the 3D model of the patient's skin surface obtained from pre-interventional CBCT imaging using a two-stage point-based registration algorithm. First, fast global registration [36] is used to coarsely align the two-point clouds, and this initial alignment is refined using an iterative closest point approach [37]. Then, this algorithm outputs the desired position and orientation of virtual content to ensure that it aligns accurately with the actual anatomy of the patient. A detailed description of the algorithm is discussed in the article by Gsaxner et al. [32].

2.2.2. User Interface

The AR system is controlled entirely with a virtual user interface (UI). Post-patient selection, fully automatic registration is initiated by examining the patient. The position and orientation of virtual content are continuously updated to account for patient movement, as well as to achieve a more precise alignment. However, in cases where a satisfactory alignment has been achieved and the patient is not expected to move (e.g., during sedation), the position and orientation of the virtual content can be established. Further manual refinement of the automatic registration is possible, which may be desirable to account for perceptual misalignments due to the individual anatomy of the user or to account for soft tissue deformations between the pre-operative CBCT scan and the intervention. The UI enables the user to switch between different registration modes, select different anatomical structures to visualize, and adjust various parameters related to content positioning and visualization. The UI is conveniently locked to the users' left hand, enabling them to bring it up anywhere simply by looking at their flat hand. Closing of the left hand locks the UI to its current position in the room.

2.2.3. Medical Data Visualization

HL 2 supports several means for adapting the visualization. Anatomical structures can be switched on and off, and the user can interactively modify several parameters to adapt the visualization to their individual preferences. These parameters include options to modify brightness, transparency, and other relevant visual settings. The complete digital workflow is illustrated in Figure 2.

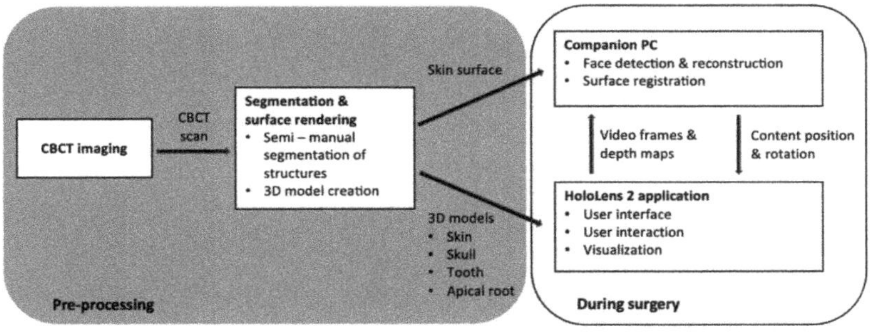

Figure 2. The flowchart demonstrates the digital workflow used in this study.

2.3. *Study Procedure*

2.3.1. Randomization

Following the selection of human cadaver head specimens, the allocation of each tooth (maxillary lateral incisor) to one of three experienced surgeons was performed using a digital randomization software (Version 2.1.0, Institute for Medical Informatics, Statistics and Documentation, Medical University of Graz, Graz, Austria; Randomizer for clinical trials: www.randomizer.at accessed on 27 June 2023) by an individual not involved in treatment or evaluation.

2.3.2. Surgery

Prior to surgical intervention, the entire tooth and the apical 3 mm of the root were marked separately and manually using data from the preoperative CBCT scan as well as 3D-Slicer® software (Version 5.4.0, Slicer Community, USA; Available at: https://www.slicer.org accessed on 27 June 2023 [38]) (Figure 3). Furthermore, the entire facial skeleton and skin surface were additionally segmented for a postliminary visualization in AR using automatic (i.e., thresholding) segmentation and manual refinement.

Preceding the trial, three experienced surgeons were given a general introduction to the HL 2 and the implemented application of virtual UI. The surgeons were given the opportunity to explore different anatomical structures and visualization modes for training purposes. Several of these training sessions took place well in advance of this study, which allowed the surgeons to become accustomed to the system, gaining both experience and confidence with its application. The outcome of this training was a reduced learning curve, minimized performance bias, and optimized study time during the actual evaluation task. Furthermore, small system-related issues could be eliminated prior to this study.

Before each surgery, the specimen was propped on the operating table, and the instruments for the procedure were prepared. CBCT imaging was registered with the patient using automatic patient registration. Certain cases involving larger soft tissue deformation between the pre-interventional scan and the specimen led to manual adjustment of the registration. Subsequently, the visualized structures and visualization parameters were adjusted for the procedure. The time to complete these preparations was logged as "preparation time", which also included a recording of the visuals.

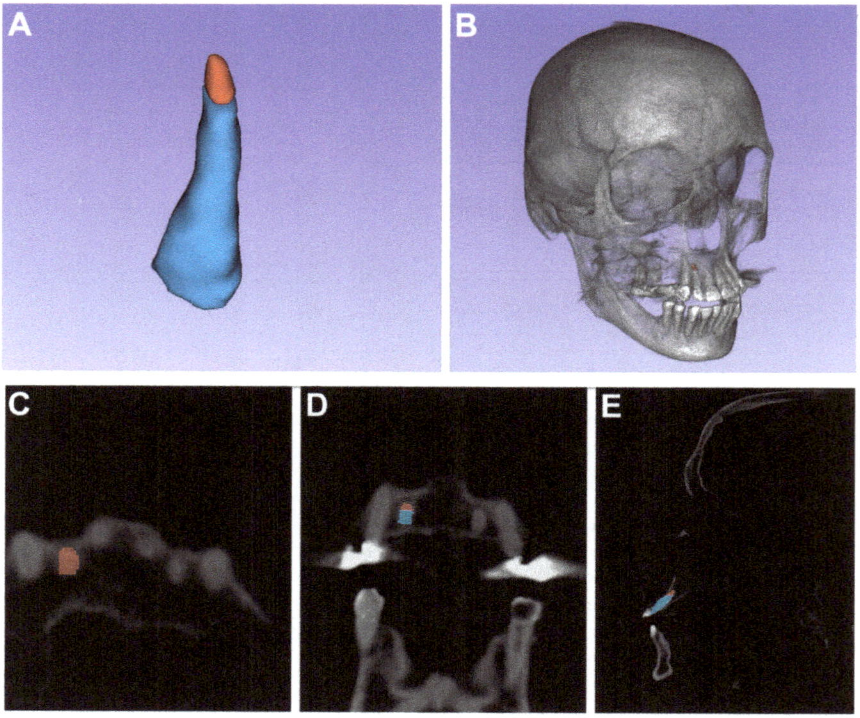

Figure 3. Preoperative rendering of the right maxillary lateral incisor using 3D-Slicer® software. (**A**): A three-dimensional model of the tooth, with the apical 3 mm of the root tip individually color-coded (red). (**B**): A model of the skull with highlighted red root tip (3 mm of the apical root tip of the lateral right incisor). (**C**): An axial plane of the cone beam computed tomography (CBCT) scan presenting the apical root tip in red. (**D**): A frontal view of the CBCT scan displaying both the root tip (red) and the root (blue). (**E**): The left maxillary lateral incisor marked in a sagittal CBCT plane.

All surgical procedures were performed following a standardized protocol at the University Clinic of Dental Medicine and Oral Health, Medical University Graz. A vertical releasing incision distally to the ipsilateral maxillary canine and a sulcular incision extending to the ipsilateral maxillary central incisor were performed with a #15 blade to create a triangular flap [39]. A full-thickness flap was raised using a Freer elevator and retracted with a surgical standard retractor. The HL 2 guidance system marked the exact spot to create a micro-invasive osteotomy using different sizes of rose head burrs to achieve exposure of the apical tip of the root. Next, a Lindemann burr was used to resect the apical 3 mm of the root tip. Thereafter, the resection surface was smoothened, and the operating field was rinsed using a physiological saline solution (i.e., 0.9% sodium chloride). Retrograde preparation and filling of the root canal were not executed. The mucoperiosteal flap was reattached with 5.0 monofilament non-absorbable single-button sutures. Figure 4 demonstrates the intraoperative setup.

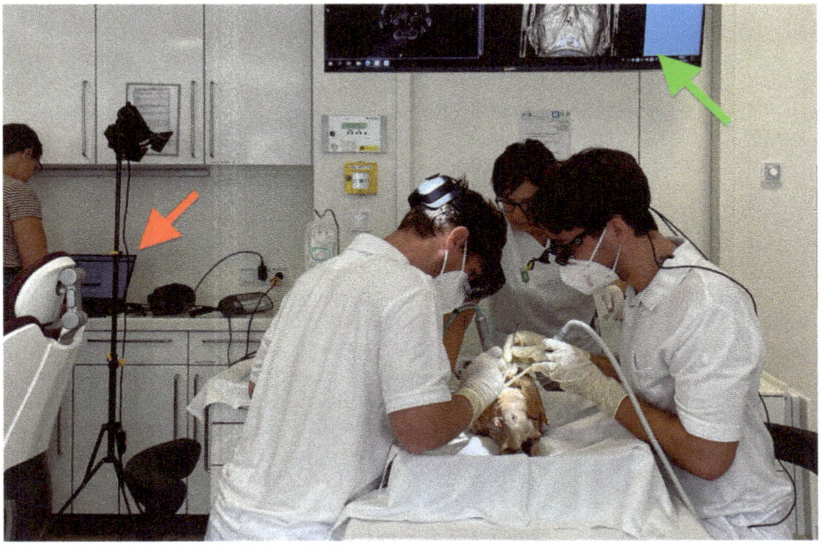

Figure 4. Intraoperative set up at the University Clinic of Dental Medicine and Oral Health, Medical University Graz. The surgeon conducts an apicoectomy on the right maxillary lateral incisor utilizing an augmented reality (AR) image guidance system based on cone beam computed tomography (CBCT) scans. The assistant utilizes illuminated magnifying glasses to optimize lighting during the procedure. A perioperative nurse provides continuous support throughout the surgery. The green arrow indicates the preoperative CBCT scans, while the red arrow marks the technical working station providing the surgeon's point-of-view. By using the HoloLense 2 as an AR image guidance system, the surgeon's focus remains completely in the operating field. With this guidance system, the need for the surgeon to alternate attention between the computer workstation and the surgical field is eliminated, allowing complete focus on the operating field by superimposing all image data (including image-based segmentation) into the field of view.

2.3.3. Measurements

For each tooth, the preparation and operating time were documented. The operating time itself was further divided into the time from incision to osteotomy and wound closure time. An accurately calibrated stopwatch was used for time measurements. Preparation time was measured in seconds, while the operating time was rounded up to minutes. These times were compared to 10 apicoectomies that the same experienced surgeons conducted prior to their AR-assisted surgeries. In order to evaluate the usability of the AR guidance system based on CBCT scans in apicoectomies, the well-established System Usability Scale (SUS) was used. The SUS is a validated, standardized questionnaire that classifies the ease of use for a wide variety of products and services such as applications or hardware. This measuring tool consists of ten items on a 5-point Likert scale [40]. Although the scores may range from 0 to 100, these values are not expressed as percentages and should be solely interpreted based on their respective percentile ranking [41].

2.3.4. Statistical Analysis

Descriptive and analytical statistics were used to analyze the gathered data, which were presented as either mean ± standard deviation (SD) or median and interquartile range (IQR). Analytical statistics included the Shapiro–Wilk test, to test the collected data for normality, followed by an ANOVA, and the Kruskal–Wallis-H test, to analyze whether there were statistical differences between users regarding setup time, operation time, and SUS score. For all calculations, a p-value of <0.05 was considered statistically significant.

All statistical analyses were performed using the statistical Python package pingouin. To additionally visualize this study's data, tables and boxplots were utilized. All specimens were anonymized before their use with the Division of Macroscopic and Clinical Anatomy at the Medical University of Graz. The recorded data were collected in a case report form. The collection, transfer, and storage of the human cadaver specimens' image data within this study was carried out in accordance with legal regulations.

3. Results

The final sample consisted of 12 teeth (n = 12) from six human cadaver head specimens (four male and two female). Each specimen underwent two apicoectomies in the maxilla, one on the left and one on the right side (24 teeth). All teeth showed no apical radiolucency in the preoperative CBCT scans. Each of the three experienced surgeons resected four maxillary lateral incisors, which had at least one adjacent tooth on both the mesial and the distal aspect to imitate structures of interest. No damage to structures of interest (e.g., adjacent roots, maxillary sinus, nasal cavity) during the procedure was observed. Throughout this study, the application encountered a singular instance of failure resulting from overheating, thus necessitating the interruption of this study until the issue was resolved using a power cycle. This incident incurred a downtime of approximately 5 min.

3.1. Times

In total, the preparation times ranged from 75 to 195 s, with an average of 162 s ± 34 s. The preparation time included automatic patient registration as well as manual adjustments (if necessary). The mean operating time was 9 ± 2 min from the first incision to the final wound closure. The fastest operating time recorded was 5 min, while the longest duration required for an apicoectomy was 13 min. Differences regarding the mean operating times among the three surgeons were not statistically significant (p = 0.940; Figure 5). Nevertheless, it is worth noting that as the surgeons gained experience with the HL, each of them demonstrated improvement in their respective operating times. The average wound closure time was 3 min 10 s ± 34 s. There was no significant difference detected among the surgeons (p = 0.681).

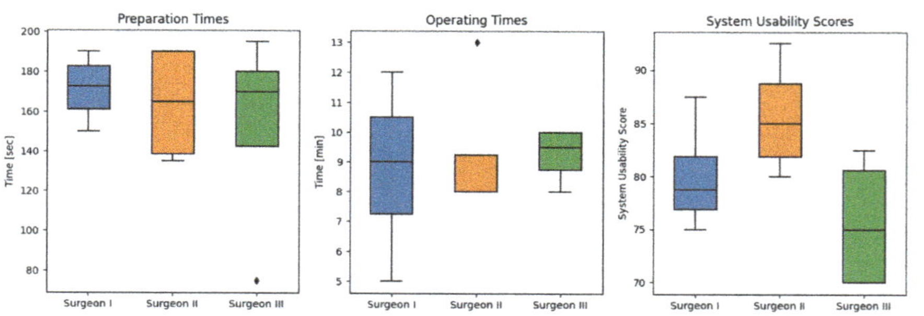

Figure 5. Box plots presenting the differences among the three surgeons regarding preparation time, operating time, and System Usability Scale score. ♦ = extreme outlier.

3.2. System Usability

The usability of the AR-guided apicoectomy based on CBCT scans was assessed using the well-established SUS questionnaire. After each surgical procedure, each surgeon promptly completed the questionnaire to assess the performance of the HL 2 based on the specific surgery that had been performed. The three operating surgeons rated the AR application with a mean SUS score of 80.4 ± 6.8, which, according to Brooke's findings [40], indicates a usability level above average (>68). The results of the used SUS questionnaires are presented as plots in Figure 5; means ± SD and median values are shown in Table 1.

Table 1. Analyzed mean and median values of the applied System Usability Scale are shown. The System Usability Scale was used by the three operating surgeons to assess the performance of the HoloLense 2 in augmented reality-guided apicoectomy procedures.

	Mean (±SD)	Median
Surgeon I	80.00 (±5.54)	78.75
Surgeon II	85.63 (±5.54)	85.00
Surgeon III	75.63 (±6.57)	75.00
Overall	80.42 (±6.81)	80.00

4. Discussion

The aim of the current study was to evaluate the intraoperative feasibility and usability of an AR image guidance system based on CBCT scans. Therefore, 24 apicoectomy procedures were performed using the HL 2 by three experienced surgeons. The evaluation of the proposed system was performed with the widely recognized SUS. Operating times were additionally measured and compared.

Apicoectomy is an approved treatment option used to preserve endodontically pretreated teeth and has demonstrated a favorable success rate [5,42]. Above all, the implementation of modern techniques like CBCT scans led to an improved diagnosis, root-end resection with minimal to no bevel, retrograde preparation using ultrasonic retro-tips, and the aid of a dental operating microscope, which have substantially improved the success rate [43,44]. Despite the promising outcome rates of the procedure, it is not exempt from inherent challenges. Protection of critical anatomical structures (e.g., maxillary sinus, mandible nerve) and accurate localization of the apical region of the root are among the most challenging steps [10,45]. Particularly, the presence of anatomical variations in tooth roots can give rise to complexities, leading to prolonged operating times, an elevated risk of inadvertent damage to adjacent structures, and prolonged wound healing due to enlarged osteotomies [46].

In order to bypass these difficulties, a variety of different navigation techniques were introduced in the past. These techniques can be roughly divided into static (SN) and dynamic navigation (DN). SN uses presurgical fabricated templates to provide guidance during the osteotomy and root-end resection. Compared with the free-hand technique, this approach has demonstrated a more precise method for accessing the apical portion of the root [8,9,47]. However, the surgical guides must be planned and fabricated in advance, which incurs notable expenses, and they cannot be modified during the procedure. Moreover, rigid anatomical structures (e.g., teeth) are necessary to stabilize the template within the oral cavity to ensure its secure position and minimize potential mobility. The utilization of a rigid surgical template presents various limitations, including impeded visualization of the surgical site, increased heat generation during osteotomy due to diminished contact of cooling fluids with the drills, and restricted mouth opening [19]. In comparison, DN shares similarities with a positioning system comprising basic equipment such as a stereoscopic camera, a computer platform with a screen, and the corresponding navigation software [10]. DN systems for apicoectomies have also been compared with the free-hand method and have shown superior results regarding accuracy and efficiency [9,48–50]. Yet, DN faces limitations. In addition to a complex assembly and a time lag for processing commands, DN forces the surgeon to divide their attention between the patient and the navigation system, while effectively coordinating the manipulation of surgical instruments [10,50].

With a head-mounted semi-transparent display in front of the users' eyes, AR can solve this attention deficit with in situ visualization [17]. Preoperative imaging has long been a standard procedure in surgical interventions. Nevertheless, surgeons face shortcomings when using these techniques. They are, for instance, forced to assess 3D imaging on 2D screens and apply this information to the patient in the operating room. The surgeon's objective is to discern the configuration of anatomical and pathological structures and estimate their size in relation to the surrounding anatomy. AR harbors the potential to seamlessly integrate radiological image data into the prevailing clinical context, superimposing it onto the patient's anatomy in real time, ensuring correct 3D alignment without any lag [20,31,51,52]. Figure 6 displays the surgeon's point of view during the surgery.

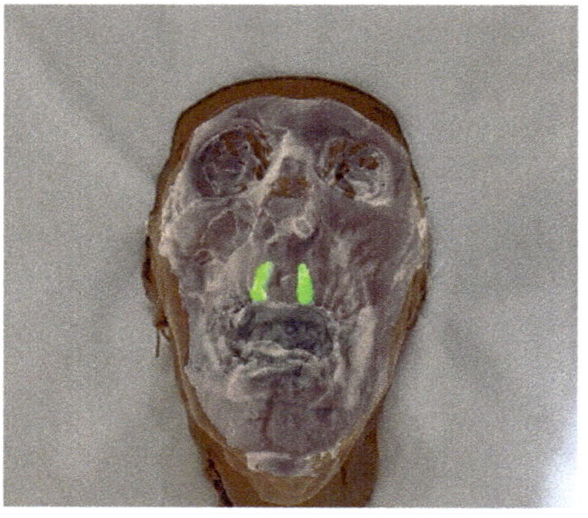

Figure 6. Superimposition of the maxillofacial CBCT scan data over a human cadaver head specimen. Hard tissue and both lateral incisors (in green) are displayed.

According to reviews by Farronato et al. and Joda et al., the predominant focus of AR in the field of dentistry lies within the context of maxillofacial surgical procedures [20,21]. Other investigated domains within dentistry include implantology, oral surgery, dental education, orthodontics, and endodontics. The frequency of studies focusing on maxillofacial surgery can be associated with the scale of the surgical field. AR systems that visualize larger objects tend to find greater applicability in this domain [46]. The most prevalent application of AR systems is in orthognathic surgery, whereby augmented and virtual reality technologies are used for prediction planning and intraoperative navigation [22]. In dental and surgical education, AR has the potential to improve learning outcomes and motor skill acquisition by integrating digital elements into the real world. Learning environments with 24/7 access and the potential objective assessment open up new teaching opportunities [21–23]. In implantology, AR mitigates surgeon-induced injuries to critical anatomical structures (e.g., mandible nerve, maxillary sinus, etc.) during the procedure and, in parallel, reduces operating times as well as error rates [18,19,22,24]. According to Chen et al., the implementation of AR in apicoectomies showed enhanced surgical precision regarding bone removal, root-end resection, and bevel angle. However, it was found to increase the duration of surgery when compared with the conventional free-hand technique. The results of the aforementioned study confirm the feasibility of an AR platform for guiding osteotomy procedures and determining apex position in an apicoectomy procedure based on a 3D-printed alveolar model. Critically perused, in this in vitro study, a "screen-through" AR approach was used; hence, the surgeon performed the operation without a direct view of the surgical field [53]. With this technique, the surgeon had to perform the operation solely based on the information gathered from a 2D monitor, which may challenge the accurate visualization of the corresponding anatomical structures, thereby potentially limiting the operating procedure. In contrast, the HL 2 AR system, used in the present study, provides real 3D visualizations of the CBCT data, superimposing anatomical structures and offering a much more comprehensive and intuitive view of the surgical field (Figure 7).

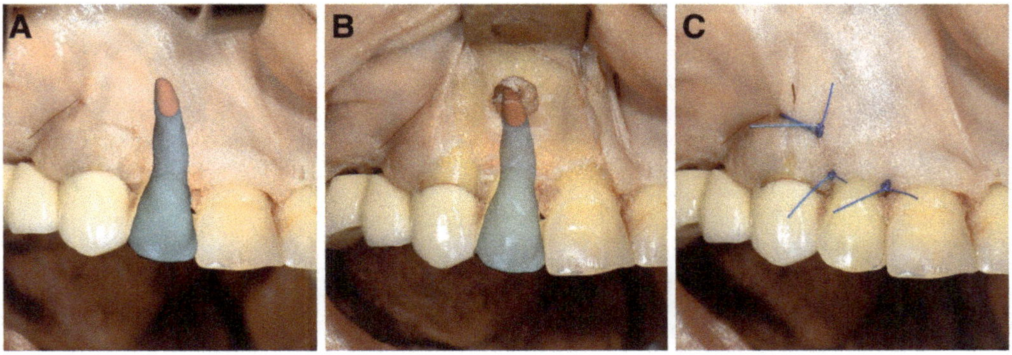

Figure 7. Real-time intraoperative views captured with the HoloLens 2 during the performed apicoectomy on a human cadaver head specimen. (**A**): The image shows a superimposed right maxillary lateral incisor model (blue) with an individually color-coded root tip (red). (**B**): An intraoperative view is shown after incision, osteotomy, and apicoectomy. The apical 3 mm of the root tip was resected according to the preoperatively planned three-dimensional superimposition. (**C**): A postoperative image showing the surgeon's perspective. The superimposition function on the HoloLens is switched off, showing only the operating field without the superimposed right maxillary lateral incisor model.

Bosshard et al. conducted a study to assess the accuracy of AR-assisted apicoectomies compared to template-guided apicoectomies using the HL 2 as a see-through head-mounted display. A favorable level of comparability between the two approaches could be shown, indicating that AR performed well in terms of medically relevant trueness and precision. Referencing the author, even a trend toward improved accuracy regarding angular deviation in the resection could be shown. Nevertheless, with respect to the time and effort required, AR assistance was found to necessitate more time subjectively due to the technical preparation involved [54]. However, in that study, the authors used a fixation technique for the pig cadaver mandibles, ensuring a stable position after registration. Additionally, a complete removal of soft tissue was performed, resulting in a simplified experimental setup. In this study, human cadaver head specimens were used to create a life-like situation while operating, which is considered an improvement to the aforementioned study design of Bosshard et al. Additionally, the specimens did not need to be positioned in a pre-determined manner. The registration process relied on an alternative system elaborated upon in the Materials and Methods section. This feature allows shortened set-up time and increased flexibility during the course of the surgery. In the present study, surgical operation times were measured and found to be comparable to in-clinic durations required to perform a conventional free-hand apicoectomy on anterior teeth, typically ranging between 5 and 8 min. For the calculation of these data, 10 apicoectomies performed at the Division of Oral Surgery and Orthodontics up to the cut-off date, the 31st of July, were collected. The mentioned 10 apicoectomies were carried out by the same three experienced surgeons. Additionally, the study team assessed the set-up time needed for technical preparation of the AR system, which was relatively low (averaging at 2 min 42 s) and would therefore not significantly prolong an operating procedure when used in a clinical case. In our user study, the presented system demonstrated above-average usability with an SUS score of 80.4 $\pm$ 6.8. Following the SUS rating system introduced by Bangor, Kortum, and Miller, this score corresponds to an "excellent" (6) system on a seven-point scale, ranging from "worst imaginable" (1) to "best imaginable" (7) [41]. Furthermore, a score above 70 indicates that the system is likely to be generally accepted by the target audience. Our study further emphasizes the equivalence in effectiveness between CBCT and the more commonly used CT scans when utilized within an AR framework [55,56]. Hence, our validation supports the potential for seamless integration of CBCT data into an AR workflow, broadening their scope of practical application to the field of dentistry.

While the presented HL 2 prototype application demonstrated its feasibility in the field of dentistry when using CBCT scans for AR-guided dental surgery, it has certain shortcomings that require attention. The current patient registration system lacks support for non-rigid registration; hence, the pre-interventional CBCT scan is assumed to perfectly align with the patient's exact appearance in situ. While the face is generally a rigid structure, this assumption may not always hold true, especially in situations like swelling, where facial features can be subject to change. In addition, structures in the lower jaw may sometimes not be reliably registered due to its mobility. The position of the mandible may differ from the pre-interventional scan, leading to small inaccurate alignments and tracking of lower jaw structures during the dental procedure. Non-rigid registration could overcome this issue. However, this is a complex process that requires real-time physics-based modeling of soft tissue properties. A further limitation is the current streaming-based approach, which incurs additional latency. The system's run-time performance becomes heavily reliant on the connection speed and processing capabilities of the companion PC, thus requiring sufficient infrastructure. As a result, users may experience delays or disruptions in the AR application's functionality. An optimized local processing-based solution, potentially available in the near future, could be a viable alternative to mitigate these concerns. The HL 2 hardware, however, cannot cater to increasing hardware requirements.

Since the adoption of AR systems in dentistry, their potential applications have witnessed exponential growth [57]. Nevertheless, several challenges remain to be addressed before these AR systems can attain widespread commercial use. In the context of surgery, the primary objective of AR systems is to enhance procedural precision. While the software has achieved considerable advancement, the central emphasis should now be directed toward augmenting hardware and technological elements to further optimize AR system performance. In dentistry, the field of operation is often confined to a few millimeters. Under static conditions, and with meticulous calibration, AR overlays exhibit exceptional performance. However, ensuring such optimal scenarios throughout surgical procedures becomes inherently complex. The dynamic nature of a surgeon's constantly moving head, as well as the patient's movements, presents significant challenges to the AR system's seamless functionality. Still, anticipating the availability of increasingly efficient mobile hardware, we optimistically foresee that these challenges can be effectively surmounted with relative ease. The inherent appeal of utilizing AR in oral surgery arises from the predominant focus on bone tissue, which is routinely assessed using CBCT scan analysis, during most surgical interventions. Moreover, the structures necessitating protection, such as the maxillary sinus, adjacent teeth, and mandible nerve, remain stable and resistant to displacement caused by soft tissue manipulation, thus enhancing the compatibility of AR with preoperative CBCT imaging. Apart from the oral and dental surgical field as shown in this study, several other dental procedures may potentially also benefit from the use of AR technology. The implementation of AR technology in these non-surgical dental procedures should be investigated in separate experiments.

5. Conclusions

AR-guided apicoectomies using the HL 2 relying on CBCT scans received an excellent rating for system utilization from three experienced surgeons. The integration of AR guidance systems into routine clinical practice is becoming more accessible, especially when relying on diagnostic CBCT scans. High peri-interventional CBCT imaging rates coupled with the presence of hard tissue-bound or well-defined structures requiring protection render this novel technology highly appealing in this specialty. As technology continues to progress, AR systems are poised to revolutionize the field of dentistry, establishing new possibilities for enhanced patient care and treatment procedures.

To further prove the advantages of the AR technology in clinical routine research, the use of a prospective split-mouth design is imperative to compare the AR-guided to the non-guided method.

Author Contributions: Conceptualization, B.R., M.R. and J.W.; methodology, B.R., M.R., C.G., J.G., M.P. and J.W.; software, C.G.; validation, B.R., M.R., C.G. and J.W.; formal analysis, B.R., M.R. and C.G.; investigation, B.R., M.R., C.G. and J.W.; resources, B.R., M.R., C.G., J.G., M.P. and J.W.; data curation, B.R., M.R., C.G. and J.W.; writing—original draft preparation, B.R. and M.R.; writing—review and editing, B.R., M.R., C.G., J.G. and J.W.; visualization, M.R. and C.G.; supervision, J.W.; project administration, J.W.; funding acquisition, J.W. All authors have read and agreed to the published version of the manuscript.

Funding: This work was supported by the Austrian Science Fund (FWF) KLI 1044 "enFaced2". We also acknowledge BioTechMed-Graz and the Macroscopic and Clinical Anatomy at the Medical University of Graz as supporting institutions of this study.

Institutional Review Board Statement: This study was conducted in accordance with the Declaration of Helsinki and approved by the Ethics Committee of the Medical University of Graz (IRB00002556, re: 31-416 ex 18/19).

Informed Consent Statement: Not applicable.

Data Availability Statement: Not applicable.

Acknowledgments: The authors would like to thank the whole team at the Department of Dental Medicine and Oral Health and would especially like to mention Erika Hafner, who made the execution of the operations possible. Furthermore, we would like to thank the Division of Macroscopic and Clinical Anatomy, which provided the human specimens. We would also like to mention Isabel Sander-Segriff, who linguistically revised our work. Thank you all. Open Access Funding by the Austrian Science Fund (FWF) KLI 1044 "enFaced2".

Conflicts of Interest: The authors declare no conflict of interest. The funders had no role in the design of this study; in the collection, analyses, or interpretation of data; in the writing of this manuscript; or in the decision to publish the results.

References

1. Nasseh, I.; Al-Rawi, W. Cone Beam Computed Tomography. *Dent. Clin. N. Am.* **2018**, *62*, 361–391. [CrossRef] [PubMed]
2. Jacobs, R.; Salmon, B.; Codari, M.; Hassan, B.; Bornstein, M.M. Cone beam computed tomography in implant dentistry: Recommendations for clinical use. *BMC Oral Health* **2018**, *18*, 88. [CrossRef]
3. Setzer, F.C.; Lee, S.-M. Radiology in Endodontics. *Dent. Clin. N. Am.* **2021**, *65*, 475–486. [CrossRef] [PubMed]
4. Setzer, F.C.; Kratchman, S.I. Present status and future directions: Surgical endodontics. *Int. Endod. J.* **2022**, *55* (Suppl. S4), 1020–1058. [CrossRef] [PubMed]
5. Truschnegg, A.; Rugani, P.; Kirnbauer, B.; Kqiku, L.; Jakse, N.; Kirmeier, R. Long-term Follow-up for Apical Microsurgery of Teeth with Core and Post Restorations. *J. Endod.* **2020**, *46*, 178–183. [CrossRef]
6. Çalışkan, M.K.; Kaval, M.E.; Tekin, U.; Ünal, T. Radiographic and histological evaluation of persistent periapical lesions associated with endodontic failures after apical microsurgery. *Int. Endod. J.* **2016**, *49*, 1011–1019. [CrossRef]
7. Setzer, F. Possible Causes for Failure of Endodontic Surgery—A Retrospective Series of 20 Resurgery Cases. *Eur. Endod. J.* **2021**, *6*, 235–241. [CrossRef]
8. Zubizarreta-Macho, Á.; Castillo-Amature, C.; Montiel-Company, J.M.; Mena-Álvarez, J. Efficacy of Computer-Aided Static Navigation Technique on the Accuracy of Endodontic Microsurgery. A Systematic Review and Meta-Analysis. *J. Clin. Med.* **2021**, *10*, 313. [CrossRef]
9. Aldahmash, S.A.; Price, J.B.; Mostoufi, B.; Griffin, I.L.; Dianat, O.; Tordik, P.A.; Martinho, F.C. Real-time 3-dimensional Dynamic Navigation System in Endodontic Microsurgery: A Cadaver Study. *J. Endod.* **2022**, *48*, 922–929. [CrossRef]
10. Saxena, P.; Gupta, S. Static vs. dynamic navigation for endodontic microsurgery—A comparative review. *J. Oral Biol. Craniofacial Res.* **2022**, *12*, 410–412.
11. Hansen, C.; Black, D.; Lange, C.; Rieber, F.; Lamadé, W.; Donati, M.; Oldhafer, K.J.; Hahn, H.K. Auditory support for resection guidance in navigated liver surgery. *Int. J. Med. Robot. Comput. Assist. Surg.* **2013**, *9*, 36–43. [CrossRef] [PubMed]
12. Manzey, D.; Röttger, S.; Bahner-Heyne, J.E.; Schulze-Kissing, D.; Dietz, A.; Meixensberger, J.; Strauss, G. Image-guided navigation: The surgeon's perspective on performance consequences and human factors issues. *Int. J. Med. Robot* **2009**, *5*, 297–308. [CrossRef] [PubMed]

13. Landaeta-Quinones, C.G.; Hernandez, N.; Zarroug, N.K. Computer-Assisted Surgery: Applications in Dentistry and Oral and Maxillofacial Surgery. *Dent. Clin. N. Am.* **2018**, *62*, 403–420. [CrossRef] [PubMed]
14. Novelli, G.; Moretti, M.; Meazzini, M.C.; Cassé, C.M.A.; Mazzoleni, F.; Sozzi, D. Introduction to Surgical Navigation in Oral Surgery: A Case-Series. *Oral* **2023**, *3*, 146–154. [CrossRef]
15. Eckert, M.; Volmerg, J.S.; Friedrich, C.M. Augmented Reality in Medicine: Systematic and Bibliographic Review. *JMIR mHealth uHealth* **2019**, *7*, e10967. [CrossRef]
16. Chen, L.; Day, T.W.; Tang, W.; John, N.W. Recent Developments and Future Challenges in Medical Mixed Reality. In Proceedings of the 2017 IEEE International Symposium on Mixed and Augmented Reality (ISMAR), Nantes, France, 9–13 October 2017; pp. 123–135.
17. Gsaxner, C.; Eck, U.; Schmalstieg, D.; Navab, N.; Egger, J. Augmented reality in oral and maxillofacial surgery. In *Computer-Aided Oral and Maxillofacial Surgery*; Academic Press: Cambridge, MA, USA, 2021; pp. 107–139.
18. Pellegrino, G.; Mangano, C.; Mangano, R.; Ferri, A.; Taraschi, V.; Marchetti, C. Augmented reality for dental implantology: A pilot clinical report of two cases. *BMC Oral Health* **2019**, *19*, 158. [CrossRef]
19. Mai, H.-N.; Dam, V.V.; Lee, D.-H. Accuracy of Augmented Reality–Assisted Navigation in Dental Implant Surgery: Systematic Review and Meta-analysis. *J. Med. Internet Res.* **2023**, *25*, e42040. [CrossRef]
20. Farronato, M.; Maspero, C.; Lanteri, V.; Fama, A.; Ferrati, F.; Pettenuzzo, A.; Farronato, D. Current state of the art in the use of augmented reality in dentistry: A systematic review of the literature. *BMC Oral Health* **2019**, *19*, 135. [CrossRef]
21. Joda, T.; Gallucci, G.; Wismeijer, D.; Zitzmann, N. Augmented and virtual reality in dental medicine: A systematic review. *Comput. Biol. Med.* **2019**, *108*, 93–100. [CrossRef]
22. Ayoub, A.; Pulijala, Y. The application of virtual reality and augmented reality in Oral & Maxillofacial Surgery. *BMC Oral Health* **2019**, *19*, 238.
23. Wang, S.; Parsons, M.; Stone-McLean, J.; Rogers, P.; Boyd, S.; Hoover, K.; Meruvia-Pastor, O.; Gong, M.; Smith, A. Augmented Reality as a Telemedicine Platform for Remote Procedural Training. *Sensors* **2017**, *17*, 2294. [CrossRef] [PubMed]
24. Jiang, W.; Ma, L.; Zhang, B.; Fan, Y.; Qu, X.; Zhang, X.; Liao, H. Evaluation of the 3D Augmented Reality–Guided Intraoperative Positioning of Dental Implants in Edentulous Mandibular Models. *Int. J. Oral Maxillofac. Implant.* **2018**, *33*, 1219–1228. [CrossRef] [PubMed]
25. Gsaxner, C.; Li, J.; Pepe, A.; Jin, Y.; Kleesiek, J.; Schmalstieg, D.; Egger, J. The HoloLens in medicine: A systematic review and taxonomy. *Med. Image Anal.* **2023**, *85*, 102757. [CrossRef]
26. Talaat, S.; Ghoneima, A.; Kaboudan, A.; Talaat, W.; Ragy, N.; Bourauel, C. Three-dimensional evaluation of the holographic projection in digital dental model superimposition using HoloLens device. *Orthod. Craniofacial Res.* **2019**, *22* (Suppl. S1), 62–68. [CrossRef] [PubMed]
27. Dolega-Dolegowski, D.; Proniewska, K.; Dolega-Dolegowska, M.; Pregowska, A.; Hajto-Bryk, J.; Trojak, M.; Chmiel, J.; Walecki, P.; Fudalej, P.S. Application of holography and augmented reality based technology to visualize the internal structure of the dental root—A proof of concept. *Head Face Med.* **2022**, *18*, 12. [CrossRef]
28. Blanchard, J.; Koshal, S.; Morley, S.; McGurk, M. The use of mixed reality in dentistry. *Br. Dent. J.* **2022**, *233*, 261–265. [CrossRef]
29. Song, T.; Yang, C.; Dianat, O.; Azimi, E. Endodontic guided treatment using augmented reality on a head-mounted display system. *Health Technol. Lett.* **2018**, *5*, 201–207. [CrossRef]
30. Gsaxner, C.; Li, J.; Pepe, A.; Schmalstieg, D.; Egger, J. Inside-Out Instrument Tracking for Surgical Navigation in Augmented Reality. In Proceedings of the 27th ACM Symposium on Virtual Reality Software and Technology, Osaka Japan, 8–10 December 2021; Association for Computing Machinery: Osaka, Japan; p. Article 4.
31. Gsaxner, C.; Pepe, A.; Li, J.; Ibrahimpasic, U.; Wallner, J.; Schmalstieg, D.; Egger, J. Augmented Reality for Head and Neck Carcinoma Imaging: Description and Feasibility of an Instant Calibration, Markerless Approach. *Comput. Methods Programs Biomed.* **2021**, *200*, 105854. [CrossRef]
32. Gsaxner, C.; Pepe, A.; Wallner, J.; Schmalstieg, D.; Egger, J. Markerless Image-to-Face Registration for Untethered Augmented Reality in Head and Neck Surgery. In *International Conference on Medical Image Computing and Computer-Assisted Intervention*; Springer International Publishing: Cham, Switzerland, 2019; pp. 236–244.
33. Thiel, W. The preservation of the whole corpse with natural color. *Ann. Anat.* **1992**, *174*, 185–195. [CrossRef]
34. Cabello, R.; González, C.; Quicios, C.; Bueno, G.; García, J.V.; Arribas, A.B.; Clascá, F. An Experimental Model for Training in Renal Transplantation Surgery With Human Cadavers Preserved Using W. Thiel's Embalming Technique. *J. Surg. Educ.* **2015**, *72*, 192–197. [CrossRef]
35. Liu, W.; Anguelov, D.; Erhan, D.; Szegedy, C.; Reed, S.; Fu, C.Y.; Berg, A.C. SSD: Single Shot MultiBox Detector. In *Computer Vision—ECCV 2016*; Springer International Publishing: Cham, Switzerland, 2016.
36. Zhou, Q.-Y.; Park, J.; Koltun, V. Fast Global Registration. In *Computer Vision—ECCV 2016*; Springer International Publishing: Cham, Switzerland, 2016.
37. Rusinkiewicz, S.; Levoy, M. Efficient variants of the ICP algorithm. In Proceedings of the Third International Conference on 3-D Digital Imaging and Modeling, Quebec City, QC, Canada, 28 May–1 June 2001; pp. 145–152.
38. Fedorov, A.; Beichel, R.; Kalpathy-Cramer, J.; Finet, J.; Fillion-Robin, J.-C.; Pujol, S.; Bauer, C.; Jennings, D.; Fennessy, F.; Sonka, M.; et al. 3D Slicer as an image computing platform for the Quantitative Imaging Network. *Magn. Reson. Imaging* **2012**, *30*, 1323–1341 [CrossRef] [PubMed]

39. Velvart, P.; Peters, C.I. Soft Tissue Management in Endodontic Surgery. *J. Endod.* **2005**, *31*, 4–16. [CrossRef] [PubMed]
40. Brooke, J. SUS: A 'Quick and Dirty' Usability Scale. *Usability Eval. Ind.* **1996**, *189*, 4–7.
41. Bangor, A.; Kortum, P.; Miller, J. Determining What Individual SUS Scores Mean: Adding an Adjective Rating Scale. *J. Usability Stud.* **2009**, *4*, 114–123.
42. De Chevigny, C.; Dao, T.T.; Basrani, B.R.; Marquis, V.; Farzaneh, M.; Abitbol, S.; Friedman, S. Treatment outcome in endodontics: The Toronto study—Phase 4: Initial treatment. *J. Endod.* **2008**, *34*, 258–263. [CrossRef]
43. Tsesis, I.; Rosen, E.; Schwartz-Arad, D.; Fuss, Z. Retrospective evaluation of surgical endodontic treatment: Traditional versus modern technique. *J. Endod.* **2006**, *32*, 412–416. [CrossRef]
44. Venskutonis, T.; Plotino, G.; Juodzbalys, G.; Mickevičienė, L. The Importance of Cone-beam Computed Tomography in the Management of Endodontic Problems: A Review of the Literature. *J. Endod.* **2014**, *40*, 1895–1901. [CrossRef]
45. Peng, L.; Zhao, J.; Wang, Z.-H.; Sun, Y.-C.; Liang, Y.-H. Accuracy of root-end resection using a digital guide in endodontic surgery: An in vitro study. *J. Dent. Sci.* **2021**, *16*, 45–50. [CrossRef]
46. Song, M.; Kim, S.G.; Shin, S.-J.; Kim, H.-C.; Kim, E. The Influence of Bone Tissue Deficiency on the Outcome of Endodontic Microsurgery: A Prospective Study. *J. Endod.* **2013**, *39*, 1341–1345. [CrossRef]
47. Ackerman, S.; Aguilera, F.C.; Buie, J.M.; Glickman, G.N.; Umorin, M.; Wang, Q.; Jalali, P. Accuracy of 3-dimensional–printed Endodontic Surgical Guide: A Human Cadaver Study. *J. Endod.* **2019**, *45*, 615–618. [CrossRef]
48. Tang, W.; Jiang, H. Comparison of Static and Dynamic Navigation in Root End Resection Performed by Experienced and Inexperienced Operators: An In Vitro Study. *J. Endod.* **2023**, *49*, 294–300. [CrossRef] [PubMed]
49. Dianat, O.; Nosrat, A.; Mostoufi, B.; Price, J.; Gupta, S.; Martinho, F.C. Accuracy and efficiency of guided root-end resection using a dynamic navigation system: A human cadaver study. *Int. Endod. J.* **2021**, *54*, 793–801. [CrossRef] [PubMed]
50. Martinho, F.C.; Aldahmash, S.A.; Cahill, T.Y.; Gupta, S.; Dianat, O.; Mostoufi, B.; Price, J.B.; Griffin, I.; Tordik, P.A. Comparison of the Accuracy and Efficiency of a 3-Dimensional Dynamic Navigation System for Osteotomy and Root-end Resection Performed by Novice and Experienced Endodontists. *J. Endod.* **2022**, *48*, 1327–1333.e1. [CrossRef] [PubMed]
51. Linte, C.A.; Davenport, K.P.; Cleary, K.; Peters, C.; Vosburgh, K.G.; Navab, N.; Edwards, P.; Jannin, P.; Peters, T.M.; Holmes, D.R.; et al. On mixed reality environments for minimally invasive therapy guidance: Systems architecture, successes and challenges in their implementation from laboratory to clinic. *Comput. Med. Imaging Graph.* **2013**, *37*, 83–97. [CrossRef]
52. Joda, T.; Gallucci, G.O. The virtual patient in dental medicine. *Clin. Oral Implant. Res.* **2015**, *26*, 725–726. [CrossRef] [PubMed]
53. Chen, Y.; Liu, L.; Qiu, S.; Hu, C.; Wang, L.; Li, Y.; Tan, X.; Gao, Y.; Huang, D. Application of Real-time Augmented Reality-guided Osteotomy and Apex Location in Endodontic Microsurgery: A Surgical Simulation Study Based on 3D-printed Alveolar Bone Model. *J. Endod.* **2023**, *49*, 880–888. [CrossRef]
54. Bosshard, F.A.; Valdec, S.; Dehghani, N.; Wiedemeier, D.; Fürnstahl, P.; Stadlinger, B. Accuracy of augmented reality-assisted vs template-guided apicoectomy—An ex vivo comparative study. *Int. J. Comput. Dent.* **2023**, *26*, 11–18.
55. Ma, L.; Jiang, W.; Zhang, B.; Qu, X.; Ning, G.; Zhang, X.; Liao, H. Augmented reality surgical navigation with accurate CBCT-patient registration for dental implant placement. *Med. Biol. Eng. Comput.* **2019**, *57*, 47–57. [CrossRef]
56. Dolega-Dolegowski, D.; Dolega-Dolegowska, M.; Pregowska, A.; Malinowski, K.; Proniewska, K. The Application of Mixed Reality in Root Canal Treatment. *Appl. Sci.* **2023**, *13*, 4078. [CrossRef]
57. Fahim, S.; Maqsood, A.; Das, G.; Ahmed, N.; Saquib, S.; Lal, A.; Khan, A.A.G.; Alam, M.K. Augmented Reality and Virtual Reality in Dentistry: Highlights from the Current Research. *Appl. Sci.* **2022**, *12*, 3719. [CrossRef]

Disclaimer/Publisher's Note: The statements, opinions and data contained in all publications are solely those of the individual author(s) and contributor(s) and not of MDPI and/or the editor(s). MDPI and/or the editor(s) disclaim responsibility for any injury to people or property resulting from any ideas, methods, instructions or products referred to in the content.

diagnostics

MDPI

Review

The Application of Cone Beam Computed Tomography (CBCT) on the Diagnosis and Management of Maxillofacial Trauma

Arif Rashid [1], Lee Feinberg [2] and Kathleen Fan [2,*]

[1] St George's University Hospitals NHS Foundation Trust, London SW17 0QT, UK; arif.rashid@nhs.net
[2] King's College Hospital NHS Foundation Trust, King's College London, London SE5 9RS, UK; lee.feinberg1@nhs.net
* Correspondence: kathy.fan@kcl.ac.uk

Abstract: The assessment and management of facial trauma in an acute setting is one of the core services provided by oral and maxillofacial units in the United Kingdom. Imaging is a pre-requisite for appropriate diagnosis and treatment planning, with a combination of plain radiographs and medical-grade CT being the mainstay. However, the emergence of cone beam CT in recent years has led to its wider applications, including facial trauma assessment. It can offer multi-planar reformats and three-dimensional reconstruction at a much lower radiation dose and financial cost than conventional CT. The purpose of this review is to appraise its potential indications in all anatomical areas of maxillofacial trauma and provide our experience at a level 1 trauma centre.

Keywords: cone beam computed tomography; CBCT; maxillofacial trauma

1. Introduction

Maxillofacial injuries are common, accounting for 5–10% of emergency department attendances in the United Kingdom (UK) [1]. Injuries can range from an isolated fracture to complex comminuted panfacial fractures, often with concomitant injuries in the polytrauma patient. Radiographic examination forms an integral part of the diagnosis, surgical planning, and outcome assessment of these patients. In the diagnostic setting, imaging should depict the location, extent, and degree of displacement of fractures and soft tissue damage. Traditionally, the standard of care was a combination of plain films perpendicular to one another. However, with the increasing availability of cross-sectional imaging, conventional helical computed tomography has superseded plain films, particularly in the assessment of upper and mid-third facial fractures.

Cone beam computed tomography scanners (CBCT) started development in the late 1990s for use in dentistry. Like conventional CT, CBCT can offer a three-dimensional (3D) view that plain films fail to provide. It uses a low-energy fixed anode tube, similar to that used in a dental panoramic radiograph machine, that rotates around the patient once, capturing data using a pyramidal-shaped X-ray beam. The field of view (FOV) can be adjusted to capture only the area of interest, allowing for the radiation dose to be 'as low as diagnostically acceptable' [2]. The result is a high-resolution, real-size dataset allowing for multi-planar reformats and 3D reconstruction, ideal for fracture assessment [3]. Images are of higher geometric accuracy and spatial resolution, with less scatter when compared with conventional CT [4], derived from a smaller and cheaper machine, and with reduced radiation [5,6].

CBCT is now widely used in the UK for risk assessment in lower third molar surgery. Its increased accessibility to maxillofacial units has lent itself to wider applications, namely for diagnosis and outcome assessments in maxillofacial trauma. The purpose of this article is to appraise the literature on its use in the trauma setting and to provide the author's experience of CBCT as an imaging adjunct at a tertiary referral trauma centre. We present the evidence base to support the wider utilisation of CBCT in facial trauma assessment, highlighting its specific indications for each anatomical region and its increasing use in the intraoperative setting.

2. Cone Beam CT Dosimetry and Safety in Facial Trauma

X-rays are the source of radiation used in both CT and CBCT imaging. X-rays are a type of electromagnetic radiation towards the higher frequency end of the electromagnetic spectrum. They are a type of ionising radiation, meaning that atoms become ionised when they are exposed to this radiation. This can result in subsequent damage to the DNA molecules within human cells, and the main risk in the context of diagnostic imaging is malignancy developing in the patient. Although the risks from these imaging modalities are very low, there is no safe dose, and as the dose increases, the risk increases.

The International Commission on Radiological Protection (ICRP) defines key principles of radiation protection that are carried forward into local legislation in different countries; justification and optimisation are two of these principles [7]. Justification is the idea that a patient should only be exposed to ionizing radiation if the benefit outweighs the risk of harm. The Royal College of Radiologists (RCR) states that 'a useful investigation is one in which the result—positive or negative—will inform clinical management and/or add confidence to the clinician's diagnosis' [8]. Optimization is the idea that every reasonable attempt is made to reduce unnecessary doses. Doses of ionizing radiation should be 'as low as reasonably practicable' (ALARP), with economic and social factors being considered [7]. Based on these principles, it would seem reasonable to perform three-dimensional imaging if this is likely to add confidence to the diagnosis and help ensure that the most appropriate management or surgical approach is utilised. Given that CBCT and conventional CT can both provide high-resolution imaging of the hard tissues, it seems sensible to consider the use of CBCT as a potentially lower-dose alternative in order to comply with the ALARP principle.

There are different ways in which doses can be presented. The most basic being the absorbed dose, which is measured in Grays. This simpler measure of dose considers the amount of radiation energy deposited per unit mass of tissue. This measure of dose can be readily established and can be taken as a readout from a scanner. However, it does not consider how ionising that type of radiation is, and it does not consider the radiosensitivity of the tissues. The gold standard measure of dose is the effective dose, as this considers all the above factors. This is measured in Sieverts. Given that the effective dose considers the radiosensitivity of the tissues irradiated, effective doses from imaging of different body parts can be directly compared. The effective dose can also be directly correlated with the risk of cancer induction. The risk of cancer induction from dental radiography is 1 in 15,000,000/μSv for men and 1 in 18,000,000/μSv for women [9]. Unfortunately, effective doses are more difficult to calculate and therefore are not available as a readout from a scanner, and in our case, we have obtained data from academic publications.

Doses for both CT and CBCT will be variable depending on the equipment used and exposure factors selected. However, a meta-analysis of published data, which included nine CBCT units, showed an average effective dose (μSv) for an adult to be 212 μSv for large FOVs. A large field of view CBCT is classified as a volume greater than 15 cm in height, therefore imaging the full maxillofacial skeleton [10]. Whereas when imaging a similar field of view with CT, an effective dose of 860 μSv was produced in another study by the same author [11]. In a further study, a range of 685 μSv to 1410 μSv was shown for CT imaging [12]. Therefore, CT imaging is, in many cases, four or five times the dose of CBCT imaging of the same anatomy.

In our institution, full-face imaging can be obtained with CBCT for a dose of around 80 μSv [13], which is potentially one tenth of the dose of CT. However, there must still be a justification for using CBCT imaging, as doses are still higher compared to conventional 2D radiography. The dose of a panoramic radiograph is around 20 μSv [14], and the dose of a single facial X-ray is around 10 μSv [15]. Therefore, a typical series of 2D imaging for facial trauma is 20–30 μSv (panoramic radiograph + PA mandible or OM 0 + OM 30 views), compared to around 200 μSv for CBCT imaging and 1000 μSv for CT imaging (Table 1). Therefore, although CBCT imaging offers a five-time dose advantage compared to CT, it is still around eight times the dose of 2D imaging. In many cases, this dose is justified by the significant increase in diagnosis confidence and detail for surgical planning that comes from 3D imaging.

Table 1. Effective Doses.

Imaging Modality	Effective Dose μSv
Facial X-ray	10
Panoramic X-ray	20
CBCT Full Facial Skeleton	200
CT Full Facial Skeleton	1000

Table showing the relative doses of imaging modalities in facial trauma.

3. Applications for Cone Beam CT Imaging in Maxillofacial Trauma

Hereafter, we describe the applications for CBCT in the assessment of trauma in the different anatomical areas of the face. A summative table of the key primary studies is provided in Appendix A. We also provide a concise guideline outlining the principles for selecting imaging examination methods for each region of the maxillofacial skeleton in Table 2.

Table 2. Choice of imaging according to anatomical area of interest.

Maxillofacial Injury Region	Suggested Imaging Modality
Dentoalveolar Injury	1st Line: Plain films (PA/occlusal/OPG) and clinical examination 2nd Line: CBCT if suspected occult root fracture or concomitant dentoalveolar fracture
Mandible Fracture	1st Line: Plain films (OPG/PA mandible views) 2nd Line: CBCT for comminuted and segmental fractures to allow for 3D printing and surgical planning; 3D assessment of condyle fractures; post-operative evaluation of complications with healing and metal work
Nasal Fracture	1st Line: Clinical examination 2nd Line: CBCT or CT if suspicion of naso-orbital-ethmoid fracture
Midface Fractures	1st Line: CBCT (if ambulatory and without suspicion of traumatic head injury and for intraoperative and post-operative assessment); plain radiographs (OM views) if isolated zygomatic arch fracture 2nd Line: Conventional CT if concomitant head injury
Orbital Fractures	1st Line: Conventional CT 2nd Line: MRI for detailed assessment of muscle entrapment; CBCT in the absence of eye signs for surgical planning and post-operative reconstruction assessment
Frontal Bone Fractures	Conventional CT for assessment of concomitant traumatic head injury

The table details the author's recommendation for imaging modality choices for fracture assessment for each anatomical region of the face.

3.1. Cone Beam CT for Assessment of Dentoalveolar Fractures

Dentoalveolar injuries are a common presentation to maxillofacial units, with a global prevalence of 15.2% in the adult dentition, 22.7% in the primary dentition, and a median age of 13.8 years [16]. Low-velocity injuries are more likely to cause damage to the supporting structures, resulting in luxation and avulsion injuries. Conversely, high-velocity injuries deliver higher energy to the crown of the tooth and are therefore more likely to produce crown and root fractures [17]. Occlusal and periapical plain films are the standard radiographic examinations utilised to assess these injuries. However, CBCT has been shown to be more sensitive when assessing for root and alveolar fractures and resorption [18,19]. The ability of a plain X-ray to detect a root fracture depends on the angle of the X-ray beam and the degree of separation of the fractured segments. One study demonstrated a detection rate of 30–40% with periapical radiographs, compared with a 90% detection rate with CBCT [20]. However, both imaging modalities demonstrated limitations when detecting vertical root fractures [21]. CBCT may also be better at assessing for pulp and periodontal healing [22,23] and thereby have a place for follow-up assessments.

Figure 1 is a small-volume CBCT scan of the anterior maxilla showing luxation injuries of the UR1 and UR2 with an associated alveolar bone fracture that extends to the anterior nasal spine. This cross-sectional imaging allows for a more detailed assessment of the supporting structures of the teeth, which may influence management decisions. Figure 2 is an example of root fractures demonstrated on CBCT imaging that were occult on plain films.

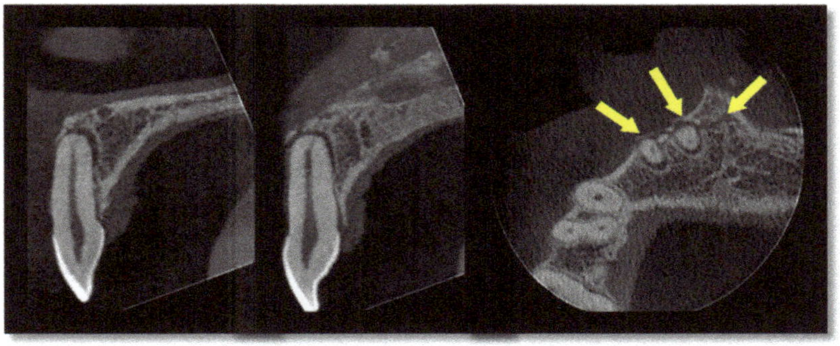

(a) (b) (c)

Figure 1. A small FOV CBCT of the anterior maxilla showing (**a**) luxation injury with (**b**) associated alveolar bone fracture (**c**) and extending to the anterior nasal spine demonstrated by the arrows.

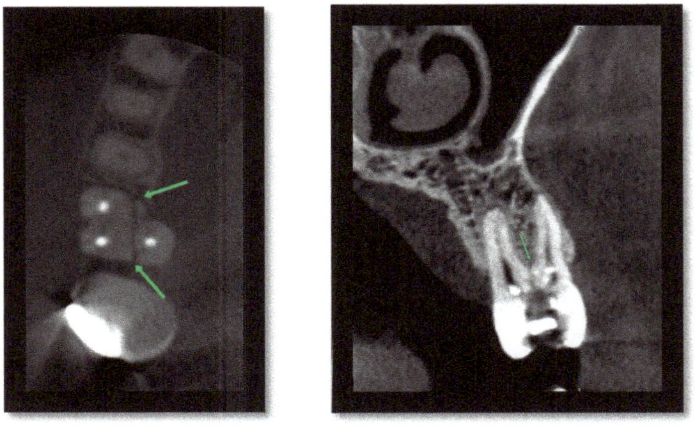

(a) (b)

Figure 2. An (**a**) axial and (**b**) coronal section of a root-treated first maxillary molar tooth demonstrating a fracture through the furcation not evident on plain films. Arrows demonstrate the fracture.

It is the author's opinion that plain films and clinical examination should remain the standard of care for initial assessment, especially as this management is time-dependent. Exceptions would include high-velocity injuries, which benefit from assessment with cross-sectional imaging. CBCT with a small FOV should be considered in these cases, especially if there is a suspected root fracture or concomitant alveolar bone fracture, in which the approach to management may be modified.

3.2. Cone Beam CT for Assessment of Mandibular Fractures

The mandible is fractured in up to three-quarters of patients with maxillofacial fractures [24]. In the demographic area served by the authors unit, interpersonal violence is the dominant cause, with the angle and parasymphysis the most commonly fractured sites, followed by the mandibular condyle [25]. Clinical examination coupled with plain radiographs (orthopantogram and posterior/anterior mandible X-ray) is often adequate to arrive at a diagnosis. The presence of a malocclusion, sublingual haematoma, step deformity, and inferior dental nerve paraesthesia can be readily assessed. Moreover, Markowitz et al. [26] found no statistically significant difference between the sensitivities for mandible fracture identification on CT compared with plain films.

Others argue that CT offers imaging-enhancing tools, improved image quality, and decreased interpretation error [27], overcoming the problems with superimposition and anatomical structure distortion in the anterior mandible and coronoid/condylar region innate to plain films. Kaeppler et al. [28] in a prospective study reported that an additional 17.75% ($n = 41$) occult fracture sites and 14.72% ($n = 34$) additional infractures were identified on CBCT (medium or large FOV was used to image both condyles), not noted on clinical examination and plain radiographs. Further information about displacement (23.8%, $n = 55$) and comminution (3.46%, $n = 8$) were also provided. In their study, this additional information, particularly occult fractures, resulted in a change in treatment in 9.52% ($n = 22$) of cases, which was statistically significant. Incomplete cortical plate fractures and their extension to the dentoalveolar segment can be better appreciated.

Condyle fractures are classified according to location (condylar head, condylar neck, subcondylar, and dicapitular) or direction of fracture (horizontal, vertical, and sagittal) [29]. CBCT offers better visualisation of TMJ anatomy, degree of fracture displacement, and comminution, which may influence surgical management. To this end, the American Academy of Oral and Maxillofacial Radiology published a position paper in 1997 [30], recommending cross-sectional imaging only in complex condylar fractures. Raustia et al. [31] found that both the antero-posterior and medio-lateral displacement of the fracture were better visualised on cross-sectional imaging. Similarly, Orhan et al. [32] when assessing vertical condylar fractures created on cadaver specimens, found CBCT was far more sensitive. In cases of intracapsular fractures, some argue the benefit of magnetic resonance imaging (MRI) to assess for internal derangement that can be simultaneously treated. Wang et al. [33] demonstrated on MRI that 91.5% of condyle fractures with dislocation showed anteroinferior disc dislocation, 87.3% showed retrodiscal tissue abnormal signal intensity, and 85.6% showed joint effusion.

It is the author's opinion that plain radiographs are the gold standard of imaging assessment for simple mandible fractures. There is a lack of robust research to support the additive use of CBCT. However, CBCT may be considered for comminuted and segmental fractures, as the ability to reformat and 3D print the images will aid surgical planning and pre-operative adaptation of plates. It also has its place in condylar fractures to better understand the direction of displacement and degree of comminution. CBCT is often used in the post-operative review setting, particularly when assessing for complications from metal work or inadequate bony healing. In a recent study [34], CBCT was used to predict post-operative inferior dental nerve injury, with associations including the proximity of the fracture line to the nerve canal and interruption along the course of the nerve. This could be of benefit to consenting patients, but further well-designed and large sample studies are needed before concluding on its predictive capacity.

Figure 3 shows plain radiographs and CBCT images of a patient presenting with an infection following open reduction and internal fixation of a left angle of mandible fracture. Cross-sectional imaging in this case was able to confirm the suspicion of non-union on the plain film, as well as the lingual bone loss and periapical area associated with the LL7 apices, suggesting a loss of vitality in that tooth.

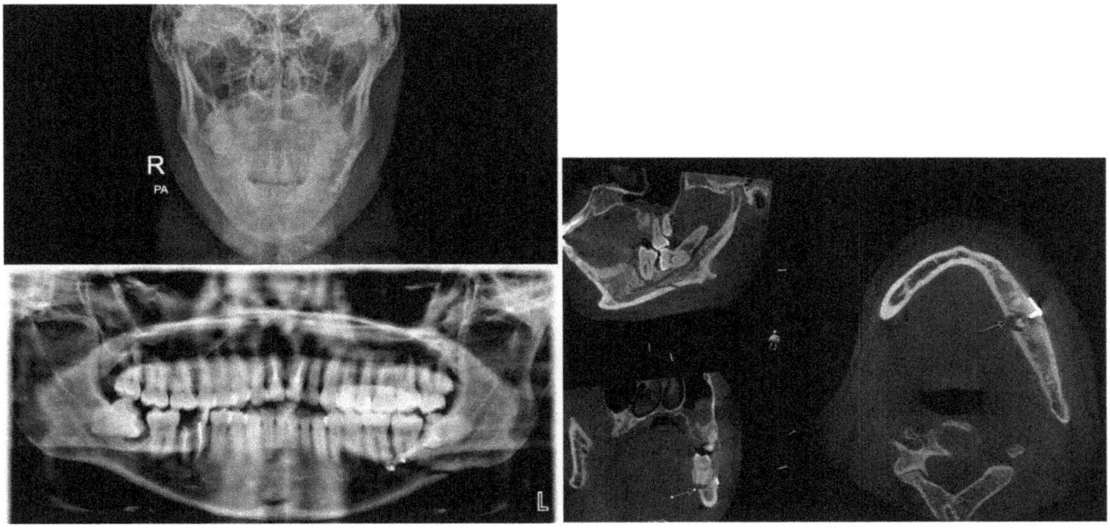

(a) (b)

Figure 3. (**a**) PA mandible and OPG and (**b**) sagittal, coronal, and axial slices demonstrating non-union of a left angle of mandible fracture. CBCT better visualizes the area of non-union and the lingual bone loss around the LL7 tooth (see arrow).

Figure 4 shows 2D images taken immediately post-operatively and CBCT images of the same patient at 24 months. The CBCT in this case can better visualise the position of the metalwork in relation to teeth and the inferior dental nerve. This added information can help inform decisions to remove metal work in patients with complications of nerve paraesthesia or non-vital teeth.

3.3. Cone Beam CT for Assessment of Frontal Sinus Fractures

Frontal sinus fractures account for between 5 and 15% of all facial fractures [35]. The most common aetiology is motor vehicle accidents. Fractures may involve the anterior or posterior table, or both, and may extend to involve the orbits, ethmoids, or nasal base [36]. They often occur with concomitant injuries, namely intracranial haemorrhage, cervical spine fractures, and other facial fractures [37,38]. For this reason, they are best investigated during the primary trauma survey with a conventional helical CT. CBCT does not provide adequate contrast resolution for assessment of underlying traumatic brain injury and therefore should not replace CT in such instances. Fractures at the level of the cribriform plate may be better visualised on CBCT, as unlike conventional CT, images are the same quality in all reformatted planes. For this reason, in a patient with persistent CSF rhinorrhoea, CBCT may be used to assess for occult fractures [39].

3.4. Cone Beam CT for Assessment of Orbital Fractures

The orbit is susceptible to injuries following blunt trauma owing to its fragile medial and inferior orbital walls. The AOCMF classification group categorises orbital fractures according to anatomical sub-regions: orbital rims, anterior orbital walls, mid-orbit, and apex [40]. Surgical exploration and reconstruction are warranted if there is muscle entrapment resulting in a functional impairment or if there are enophthalmos or hypoglobus with aesthetic implications. Non-contrast CT is the gold standard for imaging orbital injuries, providing multi-planar slices with good spatial resolution. Importantly, Ilanonkovan [41] found MRI more sensitive than CT for the diagnosis of herniation and entrapment of soft tissues, and thus MR may be utilised effectively if CT and clinical examination are not conclusive.

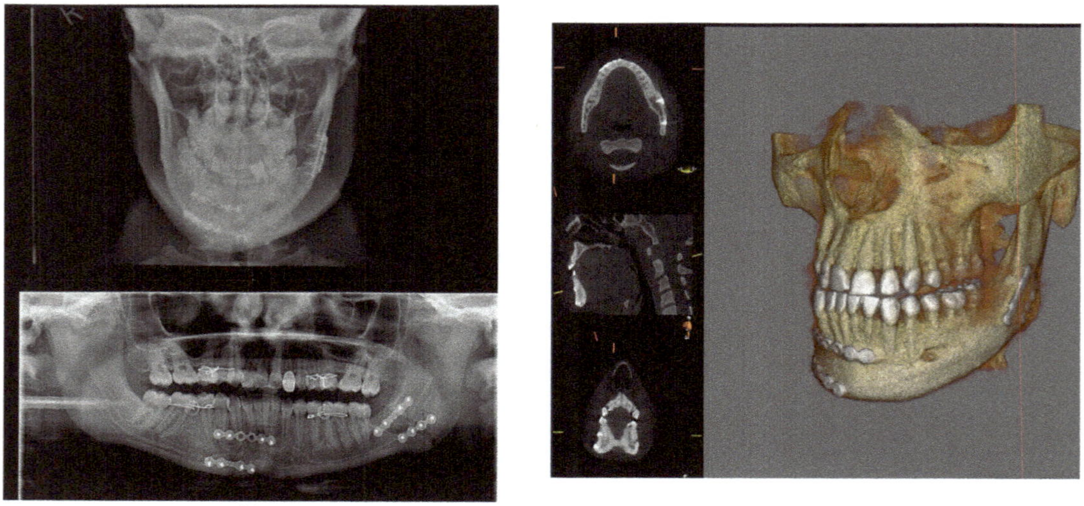

(a) (b)

Figure 4. (**a**) PA mandible and OPG and (**b**) axial, sagittal, coronal reformats, and a 3D reconstructed image. CBCT can better visualize the position of metalwork in relation to teeth and the inferior dental nerve and thus help inform decisions on metalwork removal.

The lens is one of the most radiosensitive tissues in the body, and thus, radiation to the orbits will increase the risk of cataract development. CBCT generates fewer X-ray photons, resulting in less radiation at the expense of reduced contrast. Brisco et al. [42] compared the diagnostic quality of CBCT images of orbital fractures with conventional CT. They found the soft tissue contrast was poorer in CBCT, but despite this, the imaging of the extra-ocular muscles and optic nerve was close to that of conventional CT, and entrapment was appropriately detected. However, their sample size was small, and thus caution should be taken when drawing conclusions from their results. Moreover, a retro-orbital haemorrhage was depicted in one conventional CT, but not in the CBCT of the same patient. Similarly, Roman et al. [43] evaluated 93 CBCT images of midface trauma and noted a higher sensitivity in detecting orbital floor fractures when compared with CT sections with a high level of inter-examiner agreement.

There is insufficient evidence to support the use of CBCT over conventional CT in the acute setting where there are concomitant facial or head injuries or where there is suspicion of muscle entrapment or retrobulbar haemorrhage. Figure 5 shows a CBCT coronal section of a patient with a right orbital floor fracture. The fat and muscle are indistinguishable when compared with the same slice in a conventional CT and therefore are not adequate for assessing muscle entrapment.

In the outpatient setting, in the absence of eye signs and a conventional CT, CBCT may be adequate for assessing the size of the defect and orbital volume in surgical planning. Furthermore, in this setting, mirror computational planning can be used and patient-specific implant (PSI) adapted free-hand on 3D-printed models. In the majority of cases, PSIs are acquired from conventional CT data. However, studies have shown the feasibility of using CBCT to construct orbital PSI [44]. At the time of publication, CBCT scans were not accepted for PEEKMilled implants, Titanium 3D-printed orbital and cranial implants by some medical technology companies (Synthes CMF CT-CBCT Scan Protocol) [45]. In our unit, CBCT is frequently utilised to assess the adequacy of orbital reconstruction (Figure 5).

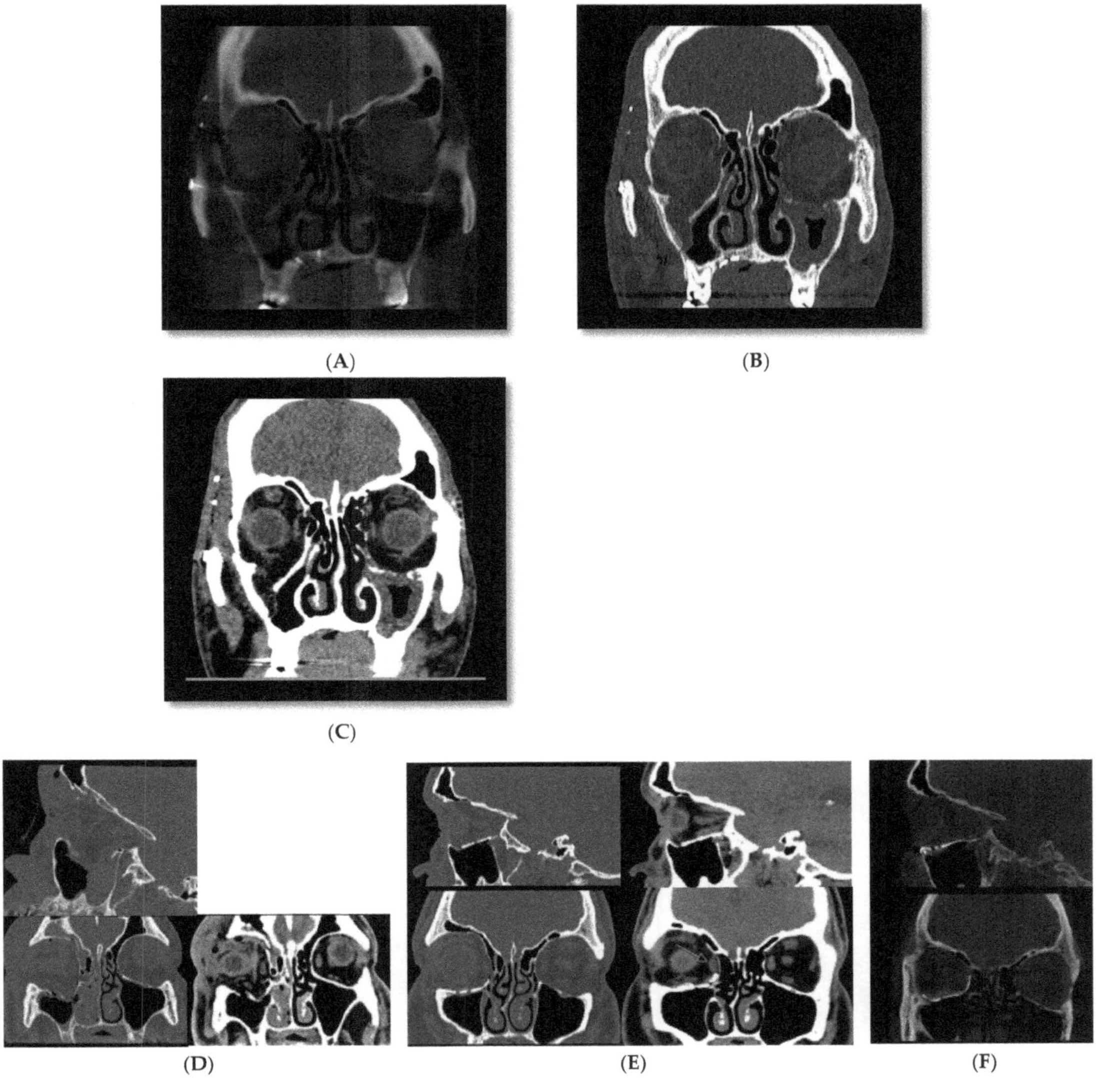

(A) (B) (C) (D) (E) (F)

Figure 5. CBCT (**A**) CT bone window (**B**) and CT soft tissue window (**C**) of the same patient, showing a right orbital floor fracture with soft tissue herniation. CT soft tissue windowing allows for differentiation between fat and muscle. On CBCT fat and muscle are indistinguishable. CBCT is suitable for assessment of the bony injury, but it is not possible to assess for muscle entrapment on CBCT. CT (**D**) at time of acute orbital trauma shows a right orbital fracture involving the floor, medial wall, and orbital roof. Soft tissue windows show inferior and medial rectus herniation. CT (**E**) prior to revision orbital floor repair shows that the medial rectus is herniating into a persistent medial wall defect (see arrow). CBCT (**F**) post-revision orbital floor repair shows that the new custom plate is well positioned with repair of both the floor and medial wall.

3.5. Cone Beam CT for Assessment of Nasal Fractures

The nasal bones are the most commonly fractured facial bones [46], owing to their central position and prominent projection. A fractured nasal bone warranting intervention is usually apparent on clinical examination, and traditionally, imaging has not been added to diagnosis or therapeutic interventions. Indeed, a patient may have a displaced nasal bone fracture clinically, but normal-appearing occipto-mental X-rays [39,47] fail to demonstrate cartilaginous disruptions or fractures.

CBCT can be employed if there is a suspicion of an associated fracture—nasomaxillary, naso-orbital-ethmoid, and floor of the frontal sinus. Coronal reformats can aid in understanding the fracture displacement and position of the septum in the absence of nasendoscopy and thereby guide instrument reduction.

3.6. Cone Beam CT for Assessment Fractures of the Zygomatic Maxillary Complex and Midface

The zygoma is the second-most commonly fractured facial fracture after nasal bone fractures. It contributes to the structure of the midface, articulating with several bones of the craniofacial skeleton, and thus fractures can be associated with significant functional and aesthetic morbidity. In the last decade, conventional CT has replaced occiptomental plain radiographs as the gold standard for imaging assessment. The ability to review imaging in multiple planes can aid the surgeon in understanding the direction of displacement to plan the reduction and fixation required for stability. Figure 6 demonstrates the difficulties with interpreting OM views owing to the superimposition of anatomical structures. The left zygomatic complex fracture is much better visualised on CBCT-reconstructed images.

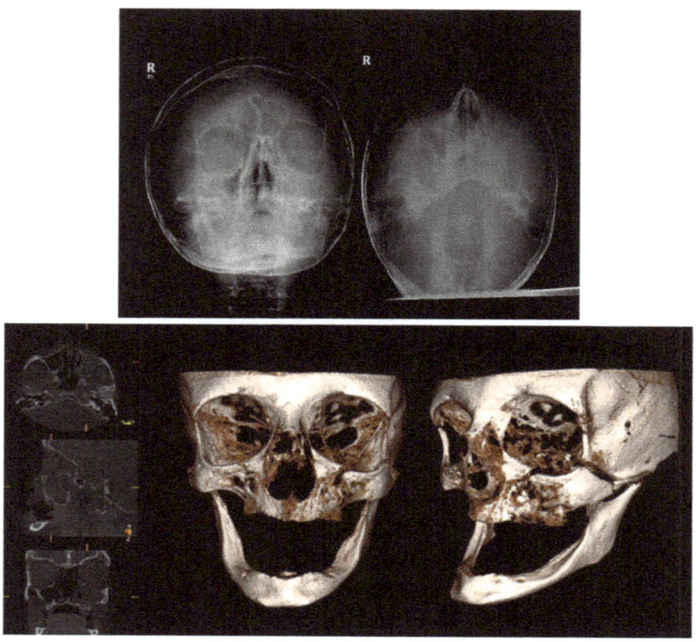

Figure 6. Occipitomental views and CBCT axial, sagittal, coronal, and 3D reformatted images demonstrating a fracture to the left zygomatic complex. Conventional occipitomental views are difficult to interpret owing to superimposition. CBCT-reformatted images show the comminuted nature of the fracture and also allow for visualization of the orbital floor.

When compared to conventional CT, a recent blinded and randomised study by Rozema et al. [48] assessed the reliability of CBCT with low-dose multi-detector CT on unilateral zygomaticomaxillary fractures on fresh frozen human cadaver specimens, demonstrating similar diagnostic capabilities. Heiland et al. [49] recommended CBCT over conventional CT in the absence of neurological symptoms or extensive injuries.

Similarly, midface fractures comprising a Le Fort Pattern are best appreciated with cross-sectional imaging. These fractures often accompany a multi-injured patient, and thus conventional CT is more readily utilised in non-ambulatory and comorbid patients. Otherwise, CBCT can show a larger number of fracture lines and fragments [40], and 3D printing can facilitate surgical planning, the alignment of teeth, and the construction of custom arch bars without the need for impressions. In our unit, CBCT is often utilised to assess fracture reduction post fixation (Figure 7). This serves as a baseline post-operative image and a more reliable assessment of bone reduction than a plain X-ray.

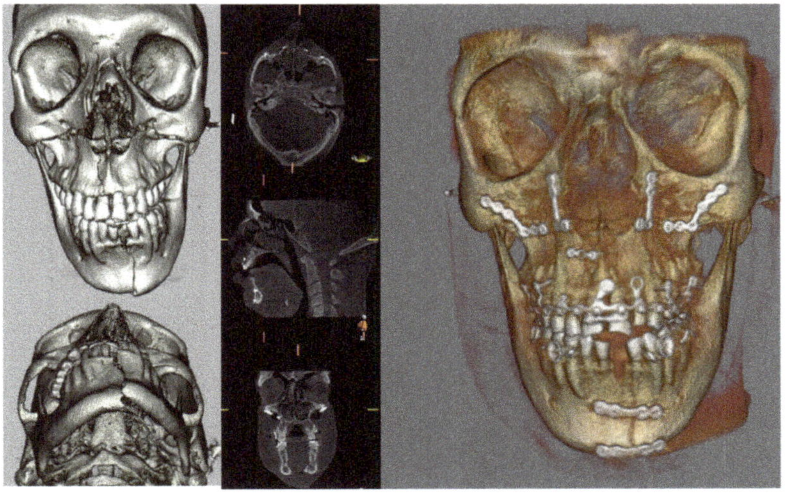

Figure 7. Pre-operative CT 3D volume renders and post-operative CBCT axial, sagittal, coronal slices, and 3D volume render showing reduction and fixation of fractures through the symphysis mandible, Le Fort 1 level, and maxillary alveolar bone.

4. Intraoperative Use of CBCT in Surgical Management of Facial Fractures

Intraoperative 3D imaging first developed prominence in orthopaedic surgery, with studies demonstrating better fracture reduction, implant positioning, and reduced need for revision surgery, particularly in cases of articular fractures or fractures in complex anatomical areas [50,51].

In the last decade, intraoperative 3D imaging has increasingly been used in maxillofacial trauma. Stanley [52] and Manson [53] published some early feasibility studies, noting that even among experienced surgeons, intraoperative clinical assessment of adequate reduction of zygomatic complex fractures or orbital reconstructions was often not confirmed by the post-operative computed tomographic (CT) scan. Intraoperative CT can allow for immediate evaluation of bony or implant positioning, thereby avoiding the risk of further surgical revision.

Pohlenz et al. [54] described the first clinical applications of intraoperative CBCT with an integrated flat-panel detector in oral and maxillofacial surgery after surgical treatment of ZMC fractures. The C-arm CBCT is considered easy to use, with fewer space requirements compared with a medical-grade CT. Additional surgical time was estimated at 8 to 30 min, including setup, sterile draping, and image review [55–57]. The current CBCT C-arm has a limited FOV of 12 cm × 12 cm × 12 cm meaning the contralateral side cannot be imaged. Assouline et al. [55] suggest merging the intraoperative data set with pre-operative imaging to achieve this comparison.

Applications include the assessment of reductions in zygomaticomaxillary fractures (ZMC) and orbital reconstructions. Surgical approaches do not allow for direct visualisation, so ZMC reduction is conventionally assessed by sphenozygomatic suture reduction and subjective assessment of facial symmetry. In a retrospective study of 48 patients with zygoma or orbit fractures, intraoperative CBCT allowed for immediate revision in 6 of the 48 cases, particularly in cases of comminution [58]. Furthermore, in seven patients, the need for orbital exploration post-ZMC reduction was deemed no longer indicated, thereby preventing unnecessary orbital exploration. This is echoed by a study on intraoperative CT at a level 1 trauma Centre in Portland, Oregan [59], where CT-guided revision rates were reported as follows: orbital 31%, Zygomaticomaxillary complex 24%, Le fort I 8%, Le fort II and III 23%, naso-orbital ethmoid 23%, mandible 13%, and frontal sinus 0%.

Other uses include assessing condyle reduction and screw fixation in relation to the inferior dental nerve [60] and intraoperative localisation of foreign bodies, particularly in the case of gunshot wound foreign bodies in close proximity to at-risk structures [61].

Although the rationale and benefit of intraoperative imaging can be appreciated, cumulative ionising radiation exposure from repeated CBCT imaging, especially if intra-operative adjustments have been made, is not without risk. Johner et al. [62] reported an average of 1.3 CBCT scans per patient, and this would correlate with the complexity of the trauma. Alasraj et al. [57] reported the highest number of revisions in ZMC cases (63.6%), and these were the only cases that required a second intra-operative scan. Moreover, despite the evidence supporting its use, a recent national French survey revealed that as little as 30% of university hospital departments and 0% of private clinics were using it, with the main indication for use being temporomandibular joint surgery or orbital fracture management [63].

5. Other Applications of CBCT in the Facial Trauma Setting

There are other applications for CBCT in the trauma setting. There is less scatter and artefact from metal compared with conventional CT, and therefore it can be used effectively when assessing facial trauma secondary to gunshot injuries [64] and for localising metal foreign bodies. It is superior to CT in detecting hard-tissue injury in the immediate locality of a high-density metal projectile. In addition, CBCT-guided removal of projectiles or metallic foreign bodies intraoperatively is associated with shorter operating times and fewer complications, including major bleeding, soft tissue infections, and nerve damage [61].

CBCT has a known application in the assessment of the airway in sleep-disordered breathing patients [65]. It can be used for geometric airway volume analysis, which can assist in anaesthetic planning ('virtual laryngoscopy') and endo-tracheal tube choice [66].

6. Limitations and Drawbacks of CBCT

The additive use of CBCT to a maxillofacial department will result in financial costs in terms of purchase, maintenance, and training. It offers lower contrast resolution when compared with conventional CT and cannot be used for measurement of Hounsfield units (HUs) [67,68]. There is an increased susceptibility to movement artefact, particularly in early-generation machines. Moreover, pathways and training in competent reporting of these images must be considered before implementing them as a new standard of care.

7. Conclusions

Radiographic imaging of the trauma patient must comply with the 'as low as diagnostically acceptable' principle. The choice of imaging should be guided by the type and severity of the injury (Table 2). A combination of plain films will remain the initial screening assessment for low-level maxillofacial trauma. Further cross-sectional imaging with the ability to generate multi-plane reformats is of benefit in select mandibular trauma and the majority of midface and upper facial third trauma. In the absence of specific indications for a conventional CT, such as a concomitant head or C spine injury, CBCT offers an acceptable alternative with less radiation exposure and potential applications to all areas of the maxillofacial skeleton. Clinicians should understand these applications and their limitations.

Author Contributions: Conceptualization, A.R., L.F. and K.F.; methodology, A.R.; software, L.F.; validation, A.R., L.F. and K.F.; formal analysis, A.R. and K.F.; resources, A.R. and K.F.; writing—original draft preparation, A.R.; writing—review and editing, A.R., L.F. and K.F.; visualization, A.R., L.F. and K.F.; supervision, K.F. All authors have read and agreed to the published version of the manuscript.

Funding: This research received no external funding.

Institutional Review Board Statement: Not applicable.

Informed Consent Statement: No patient identifiable data or images have been used in this study.

Data Availability Statement: No new data were created or analyzed in this study. Data sharing is not applicable to this article.

Conflicts of Interest: The authors declare no conflicts of interest.

Appendix A. Summative Table

Study	Research Aim	Participants	Method	Summary of Findings
		Theme One: CBCT for Dentoalveolar Fractures		
Long et al., 2014 [18]	To determine the diagnostic accuracy of CBCT for tooth fractures in vivo	Meta-analysis; 12 studies included	Quality Assessment of Diagnostic Accuracy Studies 2 (QUADAS-2) used to assess quality of included studies	• The pooled prevalence of tooth fractures in patients with clinically suspected but peri-apical radiography undetected tooth fractures was 91%. • CBCT has a high diagnostic accuracy for tooth fractures. • Caution with negative test results for endodontically treated teeth.
Sha et al., 2022 [19]	To compare the efficacy of periapical; radiography and CBCT for diagnosis of trauma to the anterior maxillary dentoalveolar region in children and adolescents	190 patients (120 males and 70 females) mean age: 11.1 years (range: 5–17 years)	Retrospective observational study. Images of patients who underwent both periapical radiography and CBCT between January 2016 and January 2020. Pairwise comparison between the receiver operating characteristic curves were performed for diagnosis of crown fractures, root fractures, alveolar bone fractures, and periapical radiolucencies.	• CBCT was significantly superior to periapical radiography for the diagnosis of root fractures, alveolar fractures, and luxations and tooth resorption ($p < 0.5$). • No significant difference between diagnosis of crown fractures and periapical radiolucencies ($p > 0.5$).
Bernardes et al., 2009 [20]	To compare 2D images with CBCT when diagnosing root fractures in the general practice setting	20 patients with suspected root fractures	Included patients who were submitted to examination by periapical radiography and CBCT; two professionals examined images according to pre-established scores.	• CBCT was better than conventional radiography in the diagnosis of root fractures.
Chavda et al., 2014 [21]	To determine whether there is a difference in the in vivo diagnostic accuracy of digital radiography and CBCT in the detection of vertical root fracture	21 unsalvageable teeth from 20 patients with vertical root fracture	Digital radiograph and CBCT images compared with visual inspection of extracted tooth under a microscope.	• DR and CBCT showed similar poor sensitivity (0.16 and 0.27, respectively), but high specificity (0.92 and 0.83). No statistical difference.

Study	Research Aim	Participants	Method	Summary of Findings
		Theme 2: CBCT for Mandibular Fractures		
Kaeppler et al., 2013 [28]	To determine the clinical efficacy of CBCT for suspected mandibular fractures and to evaluate whether findings would lead to a change in management	164 patients with suspected mandible fracture (231 sites) but equivocal clinical and 2D radiograph findings	Images were interpreted by oral and maxillofacial surgeons and treatment decisions based on pre and post-imaging were compared. Linear regression analyses were performed.	• For 4.33% of sites (n = 10), no fractures were identified. • For 63.2% of sites (n = 146), suspected diagnosis was confirmed on CBCT. • Additional fracture identified in 17.785% (n = 41) and additional infractures in 14.72% (n = 34). • Treatment plan altered in 9.52% of sites (n = 22).
Orhan et al., 2021 [32]	To investigate whether panoramic radiography and lateral skull projection images with lower radiation dose can be used instead of CBCT in the diagnosis of vertical condylar fractures	15 fresh cadaver mandibles with 30 condyles with vertical fractures created	Each condyle was imaged with panoramic, LSP, and CBCT.	• CBCT detected fractures in 100% of cases and was superior to conventional techniques.
Viveka et al., 2023 [34]	To estimate the probable post-operative nerve injury in CBCT images	Observational study; 55 consecutive participants with a mandibular fracture between March 2021 and August 2022	Preop CBCT to estimate post-operative probable nerve dysfunction. Nerve function assessed with brush directional stroke test, two point discrimination, and sharp and blunt test.	• CBCT provides additional information on the position of the mandibular canal. Risk factors include fracture line near the nerve or diversion of the course of the nerve. • CBCT was 49.15% accurate in predicting post-operative nerve injury.
		Theme 3: CBCT for Midface Fractures		
Brisco et al., 2014 [42]	Comparison of the image quality and dosimetry data for CBCT of patients with suspected orbital fractures with similar data from 3 different conventional multi-slice CT techniques	10 patients CBCT (15 cm FOV) 10 trauma patients conventional CT		• Quality of CBCT images of the orbits comparable to multi-slice CT, regardless of X-ray tube variables when displayed in bone windows. • Poorer soft tissue contrast due to scattered radiation, although imaging of the extraocular muscles and optic nerve close to that of conventional CT of the sinuses or facial bones. • Retrobulbar haemorrhage not identified on CBCT.
Roman et al., 2016 [43]	Evaluate the reliability on specific multi-planar CBCT reconstruction in orbital floor fractures	93 trauma patients CBCT examination	2 radiologist assessment of axial, coronal, and sagittal sections and also oblique coronal and sagittal sections evaluating the location of orbital fractures, size, displacement, involvement of infraorbital foramen, herniation of fat or muscle, and type of fracture.	• CBCT offered good-quality images compared with bone window sections of medical CT. • Higher detectability when using reformatted CBCT sectioning. Detection and herniation superior on CBCT oblique reconstructed images. In pure coronal view, displacement and migration measurable in less than half of cases, whereas in reformatted oblique, coronal detection in almost all cases. • Good inter-observer agreement. • Not a direct comparison of CBCT with CT due to ethical implications of double exposure.
Thiele, 2018 [44]	Investigating the feasibility of using CBCT data to design and generate customised implants for patients requiring craniomaxillofacial reconstruction		CBCT data used to generate 62 implants for 51 consecutive patients between January 2015 and December 2017.	• In all cases, implants were well fitted and no implant-related complications were detected.
Rozema et al., 2018 [48]	To assess the diagnostic reliability of low dose medical CT vs. CBCT	Unilateral ZMC fractures in 4 out of 6 fresh, frozen human cadaver head specimens	Blind; 16 radiologists and 8 OMFS surgeons performed randomised image assessments.	• ZMC fractures correctly diagnosed in 90.3% (n = 130) assessments. Dose reduction did not reduce the diagnostic reliability of MDCT and CBCT for ZMC fractures.

Study	Research Aim	Participants	Method	Summary of Findings
		Theme Four: Intraoperative CBCT		
Heiland et al., 2005 [49]	Assessment of the adequacy of intraoperative CBCT	14 patients undergoing surgical treatment for ZMC fractures	CBCT dataset generated and axial, coronal, and sagittal reconstructions evaluated by 5 examiners assessing 6 defined criteria.	• Secondary reconstructions available in 6 min. • Because of the size of the datasets, assessment of symmetry of the malar projection proved difficult. • Best-scoring results with regards to visualisation of fragment position, bony anchorage of screws and fitting of plates.
Pohlenz et al., 2009 [54]	Describe the first clinical application of CBCT with an integrated flat-panel detector for ZMC fractures	9 CBCT datasets of patients with a ZMC fracture were acquired intraoperatively using a mobile isocentric C-arm including a flat-panel detector	4 OMFS surgeons and 2 radiologists evaluated each dataset regarding noise, transition, and delineation of landmarks.	• The size of the FOV increased to allow visualisation of the whole facial skeleton.
Singh et al., 2015 [56]	Describe the use of intraoperative CBCT C arm for ZMC malpositioning	1 case ZMC malpositioning in a patient with panfacial fractures	Case report	• Intraoperative CT scan allowed for immediate revision; helpful in patients with panfacial fractures and distorted anatomical landmarks.
Alasraj et al., 2021 [57]	To determine how intraoperative CT affects the intraoperative revision rate	22 patients underwent 25 intraoperative scans	Retrospective study. Primary outcome variable: immediate revision rate. Secondary outcome: total scanning time.	• 50% required an intraoperative revision and 12.6% a repeat scan. • Mean scanning time: 18.9 +/− 4.6 min. • Highest rate of revisions in ZMC (63.6%). • None of the patients required secondary corrective surgery.
Gander et al., 2018 [58]	Assess the use of intraoperative CBCT for determining intraoperative revision rate and need for additional reconstruction of the orbit	47 consecutive patients with simple or complex ZMC fractures	Retrospective analysis. Intraoperative CBCT (Xoran Technologies, Ann Arbor, MI, USA) was overlaid on preoperative image using iPlan software (Brainlab, Feldkirchen, Germany).	• 6/48 intraoperative revisions were necessary. • Of these, 5/6 were comminuted fractures. • In 7, patients the indication for orbital reconstruction was revised.
Cuddy et al., 2018 [59]	To quantify the effect of intraoperative CT on surgical decision making	161 patients, consecutive recruitment	Retrospective case series; level 1 trauma centre.	• CT-directed revision rate: 31% orbital, 24% ZMC, 8% Le fort I, 23% Le fort II and III, 23% NOE, 13% mandible, and 0% frontal sinus.

References

1. Davies, R.; Hammond, D.; Ridout, F.; Hutchison, I.; Magennis, P. British Association of Oral and Maxillofacial Surgeons' National Facial Injury Surveys: Hard tissue facial injuries presenting to UK emergency departments. *Br. J. Oral Maxillofac. Surg.* **2020**, *58*, 152–157. [CrossRef] [PubMed]
2. Scarfe, W.C.; Farman, A.G. Cone beam computed tomography: Volume acquisition. In *Oral Radiology Principles and Interpretation*, 7th ed.; White, S.C., Pharoah, M.J., Eds.; Mosby: St. Louis, MO, USA, 2014; pp. 185–198.
3. Scarfe, W.C. Imaging of maxillofacial trauma: Evolutions and emerging revolutions. *Oral Surg. Oral Med. Oral Pathol. Oral Radiol. Endodontol.* **2005**, *100*, S75–S96. [CrossRef] [PubMed]
4. Eskandarlou, A.; Poorolajal, J.; Talaeipour, A.R.; Talebi, S.; Talaeipour, M. Comparison between cone beam computed tomography in diagnostic accuracy of maxillofacial fractures in dried human skull: An in vitro study. *Dent. Traumatol.* **2014**, *30*, 162–168. [CrossRef] [PubMed]
5. Mah, J.K.; Danforth, R.A.; Bumann, A.; Hatcher, D. Radiation absorbed in maxillofacial imaging with a new dental computed tomography device. *Oral Surg. Oral Med. Oral Pathol. Oral Radiol. Endodontol.* **2003**, *96*, 508–513. [CrossRef] [PubMed]
6. Schulze, D.; Heiland, M.; Thurmann, H.; Adam, G. Radiation exposure during midfacial imaging using 4- and 16-slice computed tomography, cone beam computed tomography systems and conventional radiography. *Dentomaxillofac. Radiol.* **2004**, *33*, 83–86. [CrossRef] [PubMed]
7. ICRP. The 2007 Recommendations of the International Commission on Radiological Protection. ICRP Publication 103. *Ann. ICRP* **2007**, *37*. Available online: www.icrp.org/publication.asp?id=ICRP%20Publication%20103 (accessed on 1 September 2023).
8. Royal College of Radiologists. *iRefer: Making the Best Use of Clinical Radiology*, 8th ed.; 2017; Available online: www.rcr.ac.uk/publication/irefer-making-best-use-clinical-radiology-eighth-edition (accessed on 1 September 2023).
9. Horner, K.; Eaton, K. *Selection Criteria for Dental Radiography Standards*, 3rd ed. 2018. Available online: www.fgdp.org.uk/selection-criteria-dental-radiography (accessed on 1 September 2023).

10. Ludlow, J.B.; Timothy, R.; Walker, C.; Hunter, R.; Benavides, E.; Samuelson, D.B.; Scheske, M.J. Effective dose of dental CBCT—A meta analysis of published data and additional data for nine CBCT units. *Dentomaxillofac. Radiol.* **2015**, *44*, 20140197, Erratum in *Dentomaxillofac. Radiol.* **2015**, *44*, 20159003. [CrossRef] [PubMed]
11. Ludlow, J.B.; Ivanovic, M. Comparative dosimetry of dental CBCT devices and 64-slice CT for oral and maxillofacial radiology. *Oral Surg. Oral Med. Oral Pathol. Oral Radiol. Endodontol.* **2008**, *106*, 106–114. [CrossRef]
12. Suomalainen, A.; Kiljunen, T.; Käser, Y.; Peltola, J.; Kortesniemi, M. Dosimetry and image quality of four dental cone beam computed tomography scanners compared with multislice computed tomography scanners. *Dentomaxillofac. Radiol.* **2009**, *38*, 367–378, Erratum in *Dentomaxillofac. Radiol.* **2009**, *38*, 554. [CrossRef]
13. Davies, J.; Johnson, B.; Drage, N. Effective doses from cone beam CT investigation of the jaws. *Dentomaxillofac. Radiol.* **2012**, *41*, 30–36. [CrossRef]
14. Feinberg, L.W.; Nixon, P.P. An update on radiation protection and the ionizing radiation regulations. *Dent. Update* **2023**, *48*, 707–709. [CrossRef]
15. Shah, S.; Uppal, S.K.; Mittal, R.K.; Garg, R.; Saggar, K.; Dhawan, R. Diagnostic tools in maxillofacial fractures: Is there really a need of three-dimensional computed tomography? *Indian J. Plast. Surg.* **2016**, *49*, 225–233. [CrossRef]
16. Petti, S.; Glendor, U.; Andersson, L. World traumatic dental injury prevalence and incidence, a meta-analysis—One billion living people have had traumatic dental injuries. *Dent. Traumatol.* **2018**, *34*, 71–86. [CrossRef]
17. Tagar, H.; Djemal, S. Oral Surgery II: Part 1. Acute management of dentoalveolar trauma. *Br. Dent. J.* **2017**, *223*, 407–416. [CrossRef]
18. Long, H.; Zhou, Y.; Ye, N.; Liao, L.; Jian, F.; Wang, Y.; Lai, W. Diagnostic accuracy of CBCT for tooth fractures: A meta-analysis. *J. Dent.* **2014**, *42*, 240–248. [CrossRef] [PubMed]
19. Sha, X.; Jin, L.; Han, J.; Li, Y.; Zhang, L.; Qi, S. Comparison between periapical radiography and cone beam computed tomography for the diagnosis of anterior maxillary trauma in children and adolescents. *Dent. Traumatol.* **2022**, *38*, 62–70. [CrossRef] [PubMed]
20. Bernardes, R.A.; de Moraes, I.G.; Duarte, M.A.H.; Azevedo, B.C.; de Azevedo, J.R.; Bramante, C.M. Use of cone-beam volumetric tomography in the diagnosis of root fractures. *Oral Surg. Oral Med. Oral Pathol. Oral Radiol. Endodontol.* **2009**, *108*, 270–277. [CrossRef]
21. Chavda, R.; Mannocci, F.; Andiappan, M.; Patel, S. Comparing the in vivo diagnostic accuracy of digital periapical radiography with cone-beam computed tomography for the detection of vertical root fracture. *J. Endod.* **2014**, *40*, 1524–1529. [CrossRef] [PubMed]
22. Andersson, L.; Andreasen, J.O.; Day, P.; Heithersay, G.; Trope, M.; DiAngelis, A.J.; Kenny, D.J.; Sigurdsson, A.; Bourguignon, C.; Flores, M.T.; et al. International Association of Dental Traumatology guidelines for the management of traumatic dental injuries: 2. Avulsion of permanent teeth. *Dent. Traumatol.* **2012**, *28*, 88–96. [CrossRef]
23. Diangelis, A.J.; Andreasen, J.O.; Ebeleseder, K.A.; Kenny, D.J.; Trope, M.; Sigurdsson, A.; Andersson, L.; Bourguignon, C.; Flores, M.T.; Hicks, M.L.; et al. International Association of Dental Traumatology guidelines for the management of traumatic dental injuries: 1. Fractures and luxations of permanent teeth. *Dent. Traumatol.* **2012**, *28*, 2–12. [CrossRef]
24. Ellis, E., III; Moos, K.F.; el-Attar, A. Ten years of mandibular fractures: An analysis of 2,137 cases. *Oral Surg. Oral Med. Oral Pathol.* **1985**, *59*, 120–129. [CrossRef]
25. Rashid, A.; Eyeson, J.; Haider, D.; van Gijn, D.; Fan, K. Incidence and patterns of mandibular fractures during a 5-year period in a London teaching hospital. *Br. J. Oral Maxillofac. Surg.* **2013**, *51*, 794–798. [CrossRef]
26. Markowitz, B.L.; Sinow, J.D.; Kawamoto, H.K., Jr.; Shewmake, K.; Khoumehr, F. Prospective comparison of axial computed tomography and standard and panoramic radiographs in the diagnosis of mandibular fractures. *Ann. Plast. Surg.* **1999**, *42*, 163–169. [CrossRef]
27. Roth, F.S.; Kokoska, M.S.; Awwad, E.E.; Martin, D.S.; Olson, G.T.; Hollier, L.H.; Hollenbeak, C.S. The identification of mandible fractures by helical computed tomography and panorex tomography. *J. Craniofac. Surg.* **2005**, *16*, 394–399. [CrossRef]
28. Kaeppler, G.; Cornelius, C.-P.; Ehrenfeld, M.; Mast, G. Diagnostic efficacy of cone-beam computed tomography for mandibular fractures. *Oral Surg. Oral Med. Oral Pathol. Oral Radiol.* **2013**, *116*, 98–104. [CrossRef]
29. Loukota, R.; Neff, A.; Rasse, M. Nomenclature/classification of fractures of the mandibular condylar head. *Br. J. Oral Maxillofac. Surg.* **2010**, *48*, 477–478. [CrossRef]
30. Brooks, S.L.; Brand, J.W.; Gibbs, S.; Hollender, L.; Lurie, A.G.; Omnell, K.; Westesson, P.-L.; White, S.C. Imaging of the temporomandibular joint: A position paper of the American Academy of Oral and Maxillofacial Radiology. *Oral Surg. Oral Med. Oral Pathol. Oral Radiol. Endodontol.* **1997**, *83*, 609–618. [CrossRef] [PubMed]
31. Raustia, A.M.; Pyhtinen, J.; Oikarinen, K.S.; Altonen, M. Conventional radiographic and computed tomographic findings in cases of fracture of the mandibular condylar process. *J. Oral Maxillofac. Surg.* **1990**, *48*, 1258–1263. [CrossRef] [PubMed]
32. Orhan, K.; Ozemre, M.O.; Koseoglu Secgin, C.; Karslioglu, H.; Kamburoglu, K.; Gur, G.; Atalay Vural, S. Comparison of panoramic, lateral skull projection and CBCT images in the detection of mandibular condyle fractures. *Cumhur. Dent. J.* **2021**, *24* 129–136. [CrossRef]
33. Wang, P.; Yang, J.; Yu, Q. MR imaging assessment of temporomandibular joint soft tissue injuries in dislocated and nondislocated mandibular condylar fractures. *Am. J. Neuroradiol.* **2009**, *30*, 59–63. [CrossRef] [PubMed]
34. Mahesh, K.; Viveka, S.; Patil, K. Probability prediction of nerve injury using CBCT images in mandibular fractures: An observational study. *J. Indian Acad. Oral Med. Radiol.* **2023**, *35*, 191–196. [CrossRef]

35. Chouake, R.J.; Miles, B.A. Current opinion in otolaryngology and head and neck surgery: Frontal sinus fractures. *Curr. Opin. Otolaryngol. Head Neck Surg.* **2017**, *25*, 326–331. [CrossRef] [PubMed]
36. Gonty, A.A.; Marciani, R.D.; Adornato, D.C. Management of frontal sinus fractures: A review of 33 cases. *J. Oral Maxillofac. Surg.* **1999**, *57*, 372–379. [CrossRef] [PubMed]
37. Banica, B.; Ene, P.; Dabu, A.; Ene, R.; Cirstoiu, C. Rationale for management of frontal sinus fractures. *Maedica* **2013**, *8*, 398–403. [PubMed]
38. McRae, M.; Momeni, R.; Narayan, D. Frontal sinus fractures: A review of trends, diagnosis, treatment, and outcomes at a level 1 trauma center in Connecticut. *Conn. Med.* **2008**, *72*, 133–138. [PubMed]
39. Shintaku, W.H.; Venturin, J.S.; Azevedo, B.; Noujeim, M. Applications of cone-beam computed tomography in fractures of the maxillofacial complex. *Dent. Traumatol.* **2009**, *25*, 358–366. [CrossRef] [PubMed]
40. Kunz, C.; Audigé, L.; Cornelius, C.-P.; Buitrago-Téllez, C.H.; Rudderman, R.; Prein, J. The Comprehensive AOCMF Classification System: Orbital Fractures—Level 3 Tutorial. *Craniomaxillofac. Trauma Reconstr.* **2014**, *7* (Suppl. 1), S092–S102. [CrossRef] [PubMed]
41. Ilankovan, V.; Hadley, D.; Moos, K.; El Attar, A. A comparison of imaging techniques with surgical experience in orbital injuries. *J. Cranio-Maxillofac. Surg.* **1991**, *19*, 348–352. [CrossRef] [PubMed]
42. Brisco, J.; Fuller, K.; Lee, N.; Andrew, D. Cone beam computed tomography for imaging orbital trauma—Image quality and radiation dose compared with conventional multislice computed tomography. *Br. J. Oral Maxillofac. Surg.* **2014**, *52*, 76–80. [CrossRef]
43. Roman, R.; Hedeșiu, M.; Fildan, F.; Ileșan, R.; Mitea, D.; Dinu, C.; Băciuț, M. The use of reformatted Cone Beam CT images in assessing mid-face trauma, with a focus on the orbital floor fractures. *Clujul Med.* **2016**, *89*, 519–524. [CrossRef]
44. Thiele, O.C.; Nolte, I.M.; Mischkowski, R.A.; Safi, A.F.; Perrin, J.; Zinser, M.; Zoller, J.E.; Kreppel, M. Craniomaxillofacial patient specific CAD/CAM implants based on cone-beam tomography data—A feasibility study. *J. Craniomaxillofac. Surg.* **2018**, *46*, 1461–1464. [CrossRef]
45. CT/CBCT Scan Protocol. For TRUMATCH^{TM} CMF Products and Services. Available online: https://www.jnjmedtech.com/system/files/pdf/195166-220315%20Synthes%20CMF%20CT-CBCT%20Scan%20Protocol.pdf (accessed on 8 September 2023).
46. Yabe, T.; Tsuda, T.; Hirose, S.; Ozawa, T. Comparison of pediatric and adult nasal fractures. *J. Craniofac. Surg.* **2012**, *23*, 1364–1366. [CrossRef]
47. Leapo, L.; Uemura, M.; Stahl, M.C.; Patil, N.; Shah, J.; Otteson, T. Efficacy of X-ray in the diagnosis of pediatric nasal fracture. *Int. J. Pediatr. Otorhinolaryngol.* **2022**, *162*, 111305. [CrossRef] [PubMed]
48. Rozema, R.; Doff, M.H.; van Ooijen, P.M.; Postmus, D.; Westerlaan, H.E.; Boomsma, M.F.; van Minnen, B. Diagnostic reliability of low dose multidetector CT and cone beam CT in maxillofacial trauma—An experimental blinded and randomized study. *Dentomaxillofac. Radiol.* **2018**, *47*, 20170423. [CrossRef] [PubMed]
49. Heiland, M.; Schulze, D.; Blake, F.; Schmelzle, R. Intraoperative imaging of zygomaticomaxillary complex fractures using a 3D C-arm system. *Int. J. Oral Maxillofac. Surg.* **2005**, *34*, 369–375. [CrossRef] [PubMed]
50. Schnetzke, M.; Fuchs, J.; Vetter, S.Y.; Beisemann, N.; Keil, H.; Grützner, P.-A.; Franke, J. Intraoperative 3D imaging in the treatment of elbow fractures—A retrospective analysis of indications, intraoperative revision rates, and implications in 36 cases. *BMC Med. Imaging* **2016**, *16*, 24. [CrossRef]
51. von Recum, J.; Wendl, K.; Vock, B.; Grützner, P.; Franke, J. Intraoperative 3D C-arm imaging. State of the art. *Unfallchirurg* **2012**, *115*, 196–201. [CrossRef]
52. Stanley, J.R.B. Use of intraoperative computed tomography during repair of orbitozygomatic fractures. *Arch. Fac. Plast. Surg.* **1999**, *1*, 19–24. [CrossRef]
53. Manson, P.N. Computed tomography use and repair of orbitozygomatic fractures. *Arch. Fac. Plast. Surg.* **1999**, *1*, 25–26. [CrossRef]
54. Pohlenz, P.; Blake, F.; Blessmann, M.; Smeets, R.; Habermann, C.; Begemann, P.; Schmelzle, R.; Heiland, M. Intraoperative cone-beam computed tomography in Oral and Maxillofacial Surgery using a C-Arm Prototype: First clinical experiences after treatment of zygomaticomaxillary complex fractures. *J. Oral Maxillofac. Surg.* **2009**, *67*, 515–521. [CrossRef]
55. Assouline, S.; Meyer, C.; Weber, E.; Chatelain, B.; Barrabe, A.; Sigaux, N.; Louvrier, A. How useful is intraoperative cone beam computed tomography in maxillofacial surgery? An overview of the current literature. *Int. J. Oral Maxillofac. Surg.* **2021**, *50*, 198–204. [CrossRef] [PubMed]
56. Singh, M.; Ricci, J.A.; Caterson, E.J. Use of intraoperative computed tomography for revisional procedures in patients with complex maxillofacial trauma. *Plast. Reconstr. Surg.—Glob. Open* **2015**, *3*, e463. [CrossRef] [PubMed]
57. Alasraj, A.; Alasseri, N.; Al-Moraissi, E. Does intraoperative computed tomography scanning in Maxillofacial Trauma surgery affect the revision rate? *J. Oral Maxillofac. Surg.* **2020**, *79*, 412–419. [CrossRef]
58. Gander, T.; Blumer, M.; Rostetter, C.; Wagner, M.; Zweifel, D.; Schumann, P.; Wiedemeier, D.B.; Rücker, M.; Essig, H. Intraoperative 3-dimensional cone beam computed tomographic imaging during reconstruction of the zygoma and orbit. *Oral Surg. Oral Med. Oral Pathol. Oral Radiol.* **2018**, *126*, 192–197. [CrossRef] [PubMed]
59. Cuddy, K.; Khatib, B.; Bell, R.B.; Cheng, A.; Patel, A.; Amundson, M.; Dierks, E.J. Use of intraoperative Computed tomography in Craniomaxillofacial Trauma Surgery. *J. Oral Maxillofac. Surg.* **2018**, *76*, 1016–1025. [CrossRef]
60. Klatt, J.; Heiland, M.; Blessmann, M.; Blake, F.; Schmelzle, R.; Pohlenz, P. Clinical indication for intraoperative 3D imaging during open reduction of fractures of the neck and head of the mandibular condyle. *J. Craniomaxillofac. Surg.* **2011**, *39*, 244–248. [CrossRef]

61. Grobe, A.; Weber, C.; Schmelzle, R.; Heiland, M.; Klatt, J.; Pohlenz, P. The use of navigation (BrainLAB Vector vision2) and intraoperative 3D imaging system (Siemens Arcadis Orbit 3D) in the treatment of gunshot wounds of the maxillofacial region. *Oral Maxillofac. Surg.* **2009**, *13*, 153–158. [CrossRef]
62. Johner, J.-P.; Wiedemeier, D.; Hingsammer, L.; Gander, T.; Blumer, M.; Wagner, M.E. Improved results in closed reduction of zygomatic arch fractures by the use of intraoperative cone-beam computed tomography imaging. *J. Oral Maxillofac. Surg.* **2020**, *78*, 414–422. [CrossRef] [PubMed]
63. Olivetto, M.; Testelin, S. Use of intraoperative 3D imaging in the maxillofacial operating room: A French national survey. *J. Stomatol. Oral Maxillofac. Surg.* **2023**, 101542. [CrossRef] [PubMed]
64. Stuehmer, C.; Essig, H.; Bormann, K.-H.; Majdani, O.; Gellrich, N.-C.; Rücker, M. Cone beam CT imaging of airgun injuries to the craniomaxillofacial region. *Int. J. Oral Maxillofac. Surg.* **2008**, *37*, 903–906. [CrossRef]
65. Shigeta, Y.; Enciso, R.; Ogawa, T.; Shintaku, W.H.; Clark, G.T. Correlation between retroglossal airway size and body mass index in OSA and non-OSA patients using cone beam CT imaging. *Sleep Breath.* **2008**, *12*, 347–352. [CrossRef] [PubMed]
66. Osorio, F.; Perilla, M.; Doyle, D.J.; Palomo, J.M. Cone beam computed tomography: An innovative tool for airway assessment. *Obstet. Anesthesia Dig.* **2008**, *106*, 1803–1807. [CrossRef] [PubMed]
67. De Vos, W.; Casselman, J.; Swennen, G. Cone-beam computerized tomography (CBCT) imaging of the oral and maxillofacial region: A systematic review of the literature. *Int. J. Oral Maxillofac. Surg.* **2009**, *38*, 609–625. [CrossRef] [PubMed]
68. Angelopoulos, C.; Scarfe, W.C.; Farman, A.G. A Comparison of maxillofacial CBCT and medical CT. *Atlas Oral Maxillofac. Surg. Clin. N. Am.* **2012**, *20*, 1–17. [CrossRef]

Disclaimer/Publisher's Note: The statements, opinions and data contained in all publications are solely those of the individual author(s) and contributor(s) and not of MDPI and/or the editor(s). MDPI and/or the editor(s) disclaim responsibility for any injury to people or property resulting from any ideas, methods, instructions or products referred to in the content.

MDPI AG
Grosspeteranlage 5
4052 Basel
Switzerland
Tel.: +41 61 683 77 34

Diagnostics Editorial Office
E-mail: diagnostics@mdpi.com
www.mdpi.com/journal/diagnostics

Disclaimer/Publisher's Note: The title and front matter of this reprint are at the discretion of the Guest Editor. The publisher is not responsible for their content or any associated concerns. The statements, opinions and data contained in all individual articles are solely those of the individual Editor and contributors and not of MDPI. MDPI disclaims responsibility for any injury to people or property resulting from any ideas, methods, instructions or products referred to in the content.

www.ingramcontent.com/pod-product-compliance
Lightning Source LLC
Chambersburg PA
CBHW062055220926
51850CB00010B/2777
* 9 7 8 3 7 2 5 8 7 5 0 2 3 *